Everything you always wanted to know about European Union health policies but were afraid to ask

Second, revised edition

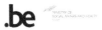

The European Observatory on Health Systems and Policies supports and promotes evidence-based health policy-making through comprehensive and rigorous analysis of health systems in Europe. It brings together a wide range of policy-makers, academics and practitioners to analyse trends in health reform, drawing on experience from across Europe to illuminate policy issues.

The Observatory is a partnership, hosted by WHO/Europe, which includes other international organizations (the European Commission, the World Bank); national and regional governments (Austria, Belgium, Finland, Ireland, Norway, Slovenia, Spain, Sweden, Switzerland, the United Kingdom and the Veneto Region of Italy); other health system organizations (the French National Union of Health Insurance Funds (UNCAM), the Health Foundation); and academia (the London School of Economics and Political Science (LSE) and the London School of Hygiene & Tropical Medicine (LSHTM)). The Observatory has a secretariat in Brussels and it has hubs in London at LSE and LSHTM) and at the Berlin University of Technology.

Everything you always wanted to know about European Union health policies but were afraid to ask

Second, revised edition

Edited by:

Scott L. Greer
University of Michigan and European Observatory on Health Systems and Policies

Nick Fahy
University of Oxford and European Observatory on Health Systems and Policies

Sarah Rozenblum
University of Michigan

Holly Jarman
University of Michigan

Willy Palm
European Observatory on Health Systems and Policies

Heather A. Elliott
University of Michigan

Matthias Wismar
European Observatory on Health Systems and Policies

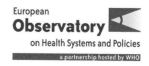

European
Observatory
on Health Systems and Policies
a partnership hosted by WHO

Keywords:

DELIVERY OF HEALTH CARE
EUROPEAN UNION
HEALTH CARE SYSTEMS
HEALTH POLICY
PUBLIC HEALTH

ISBN 978 92 890 51 767

Printed in the United Kingdom. Second printing, November 2019.

Table of contents

List of tables, figures and boxes — vii
List of acronyms and abbreviations — ix
Acknowledgements — xi
Foreword — xiii

Chapter 1: Introduction — **1**

1.1 The three faces of European Union health policy — 4
1.2 Constitutional asymmetry and the regulatory state — 7
1.3 Origins of EU health policy — 8
1.4 Three dynamics of EU health policy — 18
1.5 The emergence of a variable EU health policy arena — 23
1.6 Health, convergence and the EU — 24
1.7 Conclusion — 26

Chapter 2. The European Union: institutions, processes and powers — **29**

2.1 European political institutions — 30
2.2 Budget — 51
2.3 Strengthening legitimacy of EU health policy: civil society and stakeholders — 53
2.4 Agendas and the Sustainable Development Goals in the EU — 59
2.5 Conclusion — 62

Chapter 3. EU action for health — **63**

3.1 Public health — 63
3.2 Environment — 94
3.3 Health and safety at work — 98
3.4 Consumer protection — 101
3.5 Health systems values — 104
3.6 Health policy processes — 107
3.7 Global health and international engagement — 111
3.8 Research — 115
3.9 Conclusion — 116

Chapter 4. The EU market shaping health   **119**

4.1 Goods   119

4.2 People   125

4.3 Services   132

4.4 Competition, state aids and services of general interest   140

4.5 Innovation Union Partnership on active and healthy ageing   146

4.6 Health technology assessment   147

4.7 Trade and investment   149

4.8 Conclusion   152

Chapter 5. Fiscal governance of health   **153**

5.1 How "fiscal governance" came to exist and to matter to health   153

5.2 Fiscal governance   158

5.3 The European Semester   162

5.4 Structural funds   167

5.5 The European Investment Bank   174

Chapter 6. Conclusion   **177**

6.1 The four freedoms, constitutional asymmetry and health   177

6.2 Rethinking the EU health policy space   178

6.3 Conclusion   181

6.4 Additional reading   182

Appendices

I.   Treaty articles relevant to health today in the Treaty on European Union   183

II.   Selected articles relevant to health in the Treaty on the Functioning of the
      European Union (TFEU)   185

III. EU Charter of Fundamental Rights. Article 35 – Health Care   199

IV.   Excerpt from Mission Letter from Commission President Jean-Claude
      Juncker to Vytenis P. Andriukaitis, 1 November 2014   201

V.   Mission Letter to the Commissioner-designate for Health – Brussels,
      10 September 2019   203

List of tables, figures and boxes

Tables

Table 1.1	Impact of four different Brexit scenarios	19
Table 2.1	Order of presidencies of the Council of Ministers	40
Table 3.1	EU Member State performance against WHO tobacco control targets	66
Table 3.2	Summary of EU tobacco control legislation	67
Table 3.3	Some health impacts and associations with environmental and lifestyle factors	95
Table 4.1	Comparison between cross-border healthcare rules under the Regulation on Coordination of Social Security and the Directive on Patients' Rights in Cross-Border Healthcare	133
Table 5.1	Health-related actions in the proposed thematic objectives	173

Figures

Fig. 1.1	GDP per capita, PPP (current international $)	26
Fig. 2.1	EU budget for 2018 in relation to its GDP	51
Fig. 2.2	EU budget for 2018	52
Fig. 3.1	Major causes of death by age group in the EU25	103

Boxes

Box 1.1	EU health policies	2
Box 1.2	EU contribution to tackling cancer	6
Box 1.3	Rule of law and the EU budget	9
Box 1.4	The evolution of treaty articles on health over time	11
Box 1.5	Well-being	25
Box 2.1	Commission proposal development	33
Box 2.2	EU legislative processes	36
Box 2.3	Political groups in the 2019–2024 European Parliament and percentage of members	38
Box 2.4	Commonly used terms in EU law	42
Box 2.5	Key concepts in European integration	45
Box 2.6	Sustainable Development Goals in the EU	60
Box 3.1	International dimensions of food safety policy	78
Box 3.2	Food standards and trade agreements	79
Box 3.3	The precautionary principle	92
Box 3.4	Antimicrobial resistance	93

Box 3.5   The European Pillar of Social Rights   105
Box 4.1   International dimensions of pharmaceuticals policy   121
Box 4.2   General Data Protection Regulation (GDPR)   137
Box 4.3   Trade and Brexit   151
Box 5.1   2019 Country Specific Recommendations with reference to health   168
Box 5.2   How to read Semester documents   170

List of acronyms and abbreviations

ACTA	Anti-Counterfeiting Trade Agreement
BEPG	Broad Economic Policy Guidelines
CJEU	Court of Justice of the European Union
CPMS	Clinical Patient Management System
CSR	Country Specific Recommendation
DG DEVCO	Directorate-General for International Cooperation and Development
DG ECFIN	Directorate-General for Economic and Financial Affairs
DG ECHO	Directorate-General for Humanitarian Aid and Civil Protection
DG EMPL	Directorate-General for Employment, Social Affairs and Inclusion
DG SANCO	Directorate-General for Health and Consumer Protection
DG SANTE	Directorate-General for Health
DG TAXUD	Directorate-General for Taxation
ECDC	European Centre for Disease Control and Prevention
ECI	European Citizens' Initiative
ECJ	European Court of Justice
EFSA	European Food Safety Authority
EHIC	European Health Insurance Card
EIB	European Investment Bank
EIF	European Investment Fund
EMA	European Medicines Agency
EPSCO	Employment, Social Policy, Health and Consumer Affairs Council
ERDF	European Regional Development Fund
ERN	European Reference Networks
ESF	European Social Fund
EXPH	Expert Panel on Effective Ways of Investing in Health

FDA	Food and Drug Administration (US)
GDPR	General Data Protection Regulation
HTA	Health Technology Assessment
IMF	International Monetary Fund
IOM	International Organization for Migration
MIP	Macroeconomic Imbalance Procedure
NB	Notified Body
NICE	National Institute for Health and Clinical Excellence
OMC	Open Method of Coordination
PPP	Public and Private Partnership
QMV	Qualified Majority Voting
RQMV	Reverse Qualified Majority Voting
SARS	Severe Acute Respiratory Syndrome
SDG	Sustainable Development Goals
SGEI	Services of General Economic Interest
SGI	Services of General Interest
SGP	Stability and Growth Pact
SRSP	Structural Reform Support Programme
SRSS	Structural Reform Support Service
TEC	Treaty Establishing the European Community
TFEU	Treaty on the Functioning of the European Union
TSCG	Treaty on Stability, Coordination and Governance
UHC	Universal Health Coverage

Acknowledgements

We would like to thank Paul Belcher, Tamara K. Hervey and Olga Löblová for their generous comments and thoughts, as well as participants in a seminar with the European Commission. Errors of fact and interpretation remain ours.

Foreword

There is no European Union health system but there is an EU health policy. The EU affects the health of its citizens, the health of people around the world, and the operation and finance of its Member States' healthcare systems in many ways, mostly for the better, and often in ways that are poorly understood.

This book, a completely revised second edition of our previous volume on the subject,[1] maps out the nature of EU health policies, their logic and reason for being, and their potential to affect the health of Europeans for the better. It is written in the belief that understanding the breadth and diversity of EU health policies, and the distinctive institutional structure that explains them, will improve our collective abilities to make policy for health in any sphere, from food to healthcare services and from occupational safety to international trade.

Above all, we hope that this book makes it impossible to deny the scale and often indirect and positive impact of EU health policy. EU health policies extend far beyond the Public Health Article 168, from the environmental, social policy and consumer protection policies discussed alongside it in chapter 3, to the extensive internal market laws that have made so much beneficial EU regulatory policy, discussed in chapter 4, to the ambitious fiscal governance agenda discussed in chapter 5, which has increasingly developed a health focus. Across a broad sweep of policies from RescEU's civil protection to the regulation of pharmacies, the EU is omnipresent in health and health policy. It should be understood as such. The question is not whether we want an EU health policy, for EU health policy is inevitable. It is how it should be made and for what ends.

---

1   Greer SL et al. (2014.) *Everything You Always Wanted to Know About European Union Health Policy But Were Afraid to Ask*. Copenhagen: WHO Regional office for Europe, on behalf of the European Observatory on Health Systems and Policies.

Chapter 1

Introduction

There is no European Union health system but there is EU health policy. The European Union affects the health of its citizens, the health of people around the world, and the operation and finance of its Member States' healthcare systems in many ways, mostly for the better, and often in ways that are poorly understood.

This book, a completely revised second edition of our previous volume on the subject,[1] maps out the nature of EU health policies, their logic and reason for being, and their potential to affect the health of Europeans for the better. Almost every section has been revised and the overall structure changed to reflect changing politics and policies as well as to encourage appreciation of the extent to which the promise and potential of EU health policies lie outside the organizations, legal bases and people most conventionally associated with the health policy of the EU.

It is written in the belief that understanding the breadth and diversity of EU health policies, and the distinctive institutional structure that explains them, will improve our collective abilities to make policy for health in any sphere, from food to healthcare services and from occupational safety to international trade.

Above all, we hope that this book makes it impossible to deny the scale and often indirect and positive impact of EU health policy. Boxes 1.1 and 1.2 show the EU's impact on health and its diverse forms of influence. Box 1.1 shows how the EU is engaged in many ways in the essential functions of a health system. Box 1.2, by contrast, shows how the EU shapes one issue: cancer prevention and treatment.

This chapter maps some of the key concepts needed for understanding the EU, discussing the different faces it presents, of health policy actor, of internal market actor and of a form of fiscal governance. It then discusses the asymmetries between the EU's different roles and policy tools, and the broader range of EU powers for health that are not always appreciated by those who focus on healthcare and public health policy. This introductory chapter thereby sets up the subsequent chapters. Chapter 2 discusses the EU's institutional structure, a complex form of

---

1   Greer SL et al (2014.) *Everything You Always Wanted to Know About European Union Health Policy But Were Afraid to Ask*. Copenhagen: WHO Regional office for Europe, on behalf of the European Observatory on Health Systems and Policies.

Box 1.1   *EU health policies*

	Health legal bases				Market and wider policies shaping health				
	Public health	Environment	Health and safety	Consumer protection	Euratom	Food safety	Agriculture	Statistics	Social policy
Essential public health operations									
Surveillance of population health and well-being	X	X	X	X	X	X		X	X
Monitoring and response to health hazards and emergenices	X					X			
Health protection including environmental, occupational, food safety and others		X	X	X	X	X			
Health promotion	X						X		
Disease prevention	X	X				X			
Assuring governance for health and well-being								X	
Assuring a sufficient and competent public health workforce				X					X
Assuring sustainable organizational structures and financing									
Advocacy communication and social mobilization for health	X								X
Advancing public health research to inform policy and practice									
Domains of health systems									
Service delivery					X				
Health workforce				X					X
Information	X							X	
Medical products, vaccines and technologies	X								
Financing									
Leadership/governance									

Box 1.1   *EU health policies [continued]*

	Market and wider policies shaping health								European Semester and funds	
	Free movement – goods	Free movement – workers	Free movement – services	Research	Competition	Procurement	Taxation	Freedom, security and justice	European Semester	ESIF
Essential public health operations										
Surveillance of population health and well-being					X				X	
Monitoring and response to health hazards and emergenices										
Health protection including environmental, occupational, food safety and others	X									
Health promotion							X			X
Disease prevention										
Assuring governance for health and well-being									X	
Assuring a sufficient and competent public health workforce		X						X		X
Assuring sustainable organizational structures and financing									X	X
Advocacy communication and social mobilization for health										X
Advancing public health research to inform policy and practice				X						
Domains of health systems										
Service delivery	X	X	X	X	X	X			X	X
Health workforce		X			X			X	X	
Information			X							
Medical products, vaccines and technologies	X				X	X			X	
Financing					X		X		X	X
Leadership/governance									X	

multi-level democracy that can be difficult to compare with the Member States. Chapter 3 discusses the EU's explicit policies for health. Chapter 4 discusses EU policies affecting health that are grounded in the internal market (including some of the strongest policies the EU has in the health sphere, such as the regulation of tobacco, pharmaceuticals and medical devices), but are not grounded in health policy law and goals. Chapter 5 discusses the EU's fiscal governance system, which is still developing but contains ambitious health reform plans for Member States, far beyond what EU healthcare services policy is often understood to permit. The concluding chapter 6 summarizes the book and some of its key messages about what EU health policies are and can be.

1.1   The three faces of European Union health policy

There are three broad faces of EU health policy.[2] Each works in a different way and each is authorized by a different body of law that obliges or allows the EU to act. The first, and most obvious, face is explicit health policies, justified under the treaty provision titled "Public health" and led within the European Commission by its Directorate-General for Health, known as DG SANTE. It is a mixture of some hard powers in specific areas, such as blood products regulation, resources, notably the European Centre for Disease Control and Prevention, and programmatic activity such as the now-ended Health Programme or the State of the Health in the European Union (section 3.6.1). The treaty language that authorizes this work is clear: the organization and finance of healthcare is a Member State power, and the EU's work in public health and healthcare shall be restricted to helpful coordinating measures. This face of the EU is fully respectful of subsidiarity, the principle that the EU shall only do what cannot be done by Member States, even when there is substantial public support for more EU work to promote good health. It is nonetheless diverse and often effective, as Box 1.2 shows.

The second face of EU health policy is less intuitive to those versed in Member State health policy. It is health policy made on the legal basis of its internal market, and it is far more consequential for health and healthcare than the first face. The basic logic is that the EU has great powers to promote the development and regulation of its internal market. In particular, eliminating measures that discriminate on the basis of Member State (e.g. protectionism for one's own citizens or businesses) is a core and deeply entrenched EU power. This legal authorization means that the effective way to regulate, for example, pharmaceuticals or professional qualifications is as a part of the development of

---

2   Greer SL (2014.) The Three Faces of European Union Health Policy: Policy, Markets and Austerity. *Policy and Society*, 33:13–24; Palm W & Wismar M (2018). EU integration and health policy at the cross-roads. *Eurohealth*, 24(2):19–22; available at: http://www.euro.who.int/__data/assets/pdf_file/0009/381087/eurohealth-vol24-no2-2018-eng.pdf?ua=1

the internal market. That means both overriding discriminatory Member State regulations and raising the floor of standards so that there cannot be a race to the bottom. The result is powerful EU regulations across a range of areas, but also a persistent tendency for them to be developed with the deepening of the market rather than health as a key objective. The case law and Directive on the cross-border mobility of patients, the most visible EU healthcare policy issue for many years, was a good case: it was at every stage built around making publicly financed healthcare systems compatible with the law of the internal market, rather than promoting health or the sustainability of healthcare systems. Those issues were important for EU law and policy, not people – patient mobility is a bigger issue in EU law than for any health system.[3] In some cases, such as tobacco control, health advocates and policy-makers have had to manage legal and political complexities in using internal market rules to regulate an industry that damages health.[4]

The third face of EU health policy is fiscal governance: European surveillance of Member State fiscal policies including taxes, spending and policies that affect the state's fiscal trajectory. Fiscal governance efforts date back decades, but after the 2010 start of the European sovereign debt crisis it was greatly strengthened, becoming more ambitious, automatic and punitive in an effort to ensure that there would be no need for future bailouts because Member States would be deterred from short-sighted policies. The ambition of the fiscal governance architecture assembled in 2011–2013 is impressive, and it led to some things one might never have expected. For example, consider the 14 July 2015 Country Specific Recommendation, theoretically backed by threat of punishment, that France review its *numerus clausus* for health professionals' education.[5] That is a detailed policy intervention that few would have thought possible five years earlier. This third face of EU health policy has been evolving quickly, with debates about both its power and the ends to which it is being used. Evaluations of its actual workability and impact vary and the goals it claims to promote are broadening. The worst expectations that the strengthened fiscal governance regime would be a coercive force for austerity and health policies with no evidence base have not been proved true, in large part because the fiscal governance system and its participants have been changing quickly. Whether and when it is an effective force for better health remains to be determined.

---

3   Glinos I (2012). Worrying About the Wrong Thing: Patient Mobility Versus Mobility of Health Care Professionals. *Journal of Health Services Research and Policy*, 17:254–6.

4   Jarman H (2018). Legalism and Tobacco Control in the EU. *European Journal of Public Health*, 28:26–9.

5   Council recommendation of 14 July 2015 on the 2015 National Reform Programme of France and delivering a Council opinion on the 2015 Stability Programme of France (2015/C 272/14).

Box 1.2   *EU contributions to tackling cancer*

An alternative way of illustrating the range of EU action with an impact on health is to look at different aspects of health policy in relation to a specific disease. Here we look at cancer, as the condition with the longest history of specific EU action, across the dimensions of prevention, diagnosis and treatment, research and monitoring, and infrastructure and policy.

EU contributions to tackling cancer

For more information, see https://ec.europa.eu/health/non_communicable_diseases/cancer_en and https://ec.europa.eu/health/sites/health/files/major_chronic_diseases/docs/30years_euaction_cancer_en.pdf.

Prevention	Diagnosis and treatment	Monitoring and research	Policy and infrastructure
Primary prevention • European Code against Cancer; 12 evidence-based recommendations for people to minimize their cancer risk • Regulation of potential cancer risks in the environment (e.g.: air, soil and water quality), food safety, health and safety at work, and of tobacco products, advertising and taxation, and the creation of smoke-free environments **Secondary prevention** • Council Recommendation on population-based cancer screening and support to implementation	• Regulation of medical products, devices and technologies, such as MRI and CT scanners • Cross-border services such as tele-radiology and provision of radioisotopes • Cross-border care provision (e.g.: through European Reference Networks for rare diseases) • Cross-border care financing (e.g.: European Health Insurance Card) • Regulation of healthcare professional qualifications • Information portal for rare cancers and other rare diseases: Orpha.Net • European guidelines, e.g.: clinical guidelines on nutrition for cancer patients, and on Comprehensive Cancer Control Networks • Anti-discrimination protection for cancer patients and survivors under European legislation on disability	• Europe-wide comparative data about cancer health services and outcomes, such as from Eurostat and via cancer-specific studies such as EUROCARE and the European Network of Cancer Registries • Financing of European research on cancer • Regulation on use of personal data, for example in relation to cancer registries • Regulation of clinical trials	• Overall policy statements by the Council of Ministers and the European Parliament on cancer • Financing of cooperation between Member States on cancer, including multiple Joint Actions • European guidance on comprehensive cancer control strategies, i.e. Commission Expert Group on Cancer Prevention • Financial support to health infrastructure including in relation to cancer from the European Structural and Investment Funds, the Structural Reform Support Programme, and the European Investment Bank

As this shows, despite the primary responsibility of Member States for the organization and delivery of health services and medical care, in practice the European Union takes action in a wide range of areas that have direct relevance to cancer, which also illustrates the need to look across the full range of EU activities to understand its impact on health.

1.2   Constitutional asymmetry and the regulatory state

The EU's three faces are quite different. They authorize different kinds of action and the exercise of greater or lesser power at the EU level. The result is what scholars call the EU's "constitutional asymmetry".[6] The EU operates on the basis of what constitutional lawyers call enumerated powers: it has the powers that its founding treaties allocate to it, and no more. If the internal market treaty bases are capacious and allow extensive regulatory and harmonizing measures, then more policy will be made on the basis of the internal market. If the public health article, by contrast, emphasizes limited EU actions, then not much policy will be made on that basis. This is quite different from many federal states. For example, the broadest enumerated power the Canadian federal government has is to promote "peace, order, and good government", and this so-called "POGG clause" justifies almost any kind of social policy action. But it is not wholly determinative; the US federal government relies on its federal power to "regulate interstate commerce", the so-called "commerce clause", which is abstractly similar to the EU's internal market rules but leads to quite different public policies. In the same way, the EU's different treaty bases shape the political and organizational framing of different policy issues, the policy tools and the pressing legal issues. They do not predetermine outcomes, even if the basic mechanisms of EU law and decision-making do always lean towards the regulatory policy tool: deregulation at the Member State level and reregulation at the European.

The result of this structure is that the EU, compared to Member States, is enormously strong as a regulatory actor but strikingly weak otherwise. It is the paragon of what we call a "regulatory state", meaning a political system that acts through regulation instead of other tools such as taxation, spending and direct deployment of its own resources.[7] It regulates the actions of others, achieving public policy ends not so much through its own actions or spending as by shaping the actions and rules made by its Member States. The EU's regulatory nature explains how it can be so consequential yet in staff terms so small.[8] Its executive, the Commission, employs fewer people than many local governments in Europe. The structure of EU law means that Member State administrations implement EU law while Member State legal systems enforce it. The EU regulates Member States above all, with its legislation focused on regulating their actions and its legal system ensuring that they cannot disobey EU law. At times, this constitutional asymmetry in favour of nondiscrimination and law has actively threatened health objectives, as in challenges brought under EU law to alcohol

---

6   Scharpf FW (2002). The European social model. *JCMS: Journal of Common Market Studies*, 40(4):645–70; Scharpf FW (2010). The asymmetry of European integration, or why the EU cannot be a 'social market economy'. *Socio-economic Review*, 8(2):211–50.

7   Majone G (1994). The Rise of the Regulatory State in Europe. *West European Politics*, 17:77–102.

8   Page EC (2001). The European Union and the Bureaucratic Mode of Production, in Menon A (ed.). *From the Nation State to Europe: Essays in Honour of Jack Hayward*. Oxford: Oxford University Press.

minimum pricing (*see* section 3.1.3) or in the string of patient mobility cases in which the courts determined that health systems are a service in the single market and only later showed an appreciation of healthcare's distinctive complexity, risk pooling and social roles (*see* section 4.3.1).

EU spending is focused in agriculture, where the health effects are still not clearly beneficial overall, and in structural funds, its aid to infrastructure and development in poorer regions. These are large areas of spending, especially given their focus in a few particular countries. They are not, however, the core of EU power. The real power in the EU lies in the development of regulatory policies that harmonize standards for key products at a high level (e.g. with food safety) within an overall internal market and in a way that both Member State bureaucracies and Member State courts will implement and enforce.[9] Visible policies with supporters who will pressure Member States to comply with EU regulations become entrenched and powerful, and can shape economy and society for health.

1.3   Origins of EU health policy

The EU has affected health for as long as it or its ancestors, such as the European Coal and Steel Community, have existed. Creating and regulating markets for goods and labour necessarily involved decisions with implications for the health of workers, consumers and people in the broader environment. But health policy is always smaller and more circumscribed than it might be. In the case of the EU, and as might be expected, health was initially part of social security coordination (*see* section 4.2.2). In most EU Member States until the 1980s, regardless of their system, healthcare finance and policy were under the ministry of labour or social security rather than a separate health ministry. In the EU, correspondingly, the only healthcare issue for many years was the coordination of social security benefits that might include health. Otherwise, "public health" meant the same thing that it meant in international trade law: a possible reason for a Member State to make a policy that impeded the free movement of goods, people and services, and one that European courts regarded with some suspicion.

EU health policy as such, with health as its declared objective, began in the 1980s for fairly clear political reasons: individual heads of government, notably French President François Mitterrand, took an interest in particular health issues such as cancer. In the context of European Council meetings, Mitterrand and like-minded leaders put through commitments such as the Europe Against Cancer research programme. It was, and is, difficult to argue against agreeing to low-budget cooperation against a problem like cancer, or, later, AIDS, or harmful drug use.

---

9   Greer SL & Martín de Almagro Iniesta M (2013). How Bureaucracies Listen to Courts: Bureaucratized Calculations and European Law. *Law and Social Inquiry*, 39:361–8.

Box 1.3 *Rule of law and the EU budget*

Rule of law is a core principle of the European Union: Article 2 TEU states that "The Union is founded on the values of respect for human dignity, freedom, democracy, equality, the rule of law and respect for human rights." In recent years, as some very visible democratic backsliding has occurred, pressure has grown to police this article. The constitutional asymmetry of the EU plays out here as well: subsidiarity protects Member States, once they have joined, from sanction should they backslide. The Commission responded with a Rule of Law Framework[a] that it updated in 2019,[b] much of which was focused on identifying treaty bases to protect the rule of law in Member States. One of the most legally solid and politically promising ways to promote the rule of law is through viewing it a threat to the budget, using the logic that good budgetary governance cannot happen without rule of law. The Commission consequently proposed a Regulation "on the protection of the Union's budget in case of generalised deficiencies as regards the rule of law in the Member States"[c] that would cause the suspension of some or all EU payments to a Member State in the event that it was found to have "generalised deficiencies". Such a policy would have dramatic effects on the policies and politics of the countries that most benefit from structural funds[d] (*see* section 5.4). Note, though, the title: there is no mandate for the EU to intervene in the politics of its Member States, so it is based on the protection of the EU budget.

Discussions about the Rule of Law, a 2019 Finnish Presidency priority,[e] are not just an issue for structural funds. Commission research has found that healthcare is one of the sectors of the whole EU most plagued by corruption.[f] Expanding the effectiveness of the rule of law could have important benefits for health budgets that cannot afford corruption.[g]

[a]   European Commission. Communication from the Commission to the European Parliament and the Council. "A new EU Framework to strengthen the Rule of Law" /* COM/2014/0158 final */.

[b]   Brussels, 3.4.2019 COM(2019) 163 final Communication from the Commission to the European Parliament, the European Council and the Council "Further strengthening the Rule of Law within the Union. State of play and possible next steps".

[c]   COM(2018) 324 final 2018/0136(COD) Proposal for a Regulation of the European Parliament and of the Council on the protection of the Union's budget in case of generalised deficiencies as regards the rule of law in the Member States.

[d]   Jasna S, Bond I, Dolan C (2017). *Can EU funds promote the rule of law in Europe?* Center for European Reform.

[e]   "Strengthening the Rule of Law". Finland's Presidency of the Council of the European Union, 2019.

[f]   European Commission (2017). "Updated Study on Corruption in the Healthcare Sector – Final Report"; and: https://www.stt.lt/documents/soc_tyrimai/20131219_study_on_corruption_in_the_healthcare_sector_en.pdf.

[g]   Radin D (2016). Why health care corruption needs a new approach. *Journal of Health Services Research and Policy*, 21(3):212–14.

But, set against the rising profile of healthcare in many national polities and the rising profile of the EU in those years, it began to normalize the idea that effective European public health action was possible. That rising profile, meanwhile, was part of how the European institutions began to establish more policies affecting health. The 1986 Single European Act created the 1992 programme of market integration. It involved a long list of harmonizing measures that would mean Member States, once they had hit an EU-wide regulatory minimum, would mutually recognize each other's regulations. In these measures were some of the first European policies affecting healthcare, including the start of European regulation of pharmaceuticals and medical devices.[10]

The Maastricht Treaty was a major step forward on the trajectory of institutionalizing public health as a European power. It created, for the first time, an Article discussing public health and explicitly enabling the EU to take (limited) actions to support Member State action and cooperation on health. The concrete issues discussed in this new Article (then numbered 129) were limited and reflected the politics of the day, with action against the misuse of harmful drugs underlined as a "scourge" to be addressed. The language made it clear that there would be no major initiatives or institutional protagonism for the institutions (*see* Box 1.4).

Against the background of optimism in 1992, with the end of the Cold War, German reunification, the completion of the Single Europe Act's project, agreement on the creation of a monetary union, and talk of an ambitious "social Europe" to match the single market, the inclusion of this weak authorization for European health action should not be too surprising: it was an opportunity to do something creditworthy, might reap benefits from coordination, and had no legal language that suggested it would create a European health policy that might infringe on Member States. Its restrictive language and list of topics also put a ceiling on the European integration that had been developing apace in the form of individual disease programmes such as Europe against Cancer, so it is not completely clear that it was the step forward for health policy that it is often made out to be.

In the later 1990s more governments of the left came to power and sought to complement the preparations for monetary union with a more social dimension, creating a series of discussion forums known as the Open Method of Coordination (OMC) with the goal of pushing social policy goals such as quality services and equity onto a European policy agenda dominated by efforts to hit the fiscal goals for monetary union laid out in the Maastricht Treaty. The OMC came to include health, and while its impact on Member States' policies was indirect at best, it did start to shape shared European understandings of social policy, including health, and helped to create shared European social policy debates and concepts.[11]

---

10 Hauray B (2006). *L'Europe Du Médicament: Politique- Expertise- Intérêts Privés*. Paris: Presses de Sciences Po; Hauray B (2013). "The European Regulation of Medicines", in Greer SL & Kurzer P (eds.). *European Union Public Health Policy: Regional and Global Trends*. Abingdon: Routledge.

11 Greer S, Vanhercke B (2010). "Governing health care through EU soft law", in *Health System Governance in Europe: The Role of EU Law and Policy*. Cambridge: Cambridge University Press, 186–230; de la Porte C, Pochet P (2012). Why and how (still) study the Open Method of Co-ordination (OMC)? *Journal of European social policy*, 22(3):336–49.

Box 1.4   *The evolution of treaty articles on health over time*

Treaty on European Union (Maastricht, 1992)

TITLE XI – Consumer protection

Article 129a

1. The Community shall contribute to the attainment of a high level of consumer protection through:

(a) measures adopted pursuant to Article 100a in the context of the completion of the internal market;

(b) specific action which supports and supplements the policy pursued by the Member States to protect the health, safety and economic interests of consumers and to provide adequate information to consumers.

2. The Council, acting in accordance with the procedure referred to in Article 189b and after consulting the Economic and Social Committee, shall adopt the specific action referred to in paragraph 1(b).

3. Action adopted pursuant to paragraph 2 shall not prevent any Member State from maintaining or introducing more stringent protective measures. Such measures must be compatible with this Treaty. The Commission shall be notified of them.

Treaty establishing the European Community (Amsterdam, 1999)

Article 152

1. A high level of human health protection shall be ensured in the definition and implementation of all Community policies and activities.

Community action, which shall complement national policies, shall be directed towards improving public health, preventing human illness and diseases, and obviating sources of danger to human health. Such action shall cover the fight against the major health scourges, by promoting research into their causes, their transmission and their prevention, as well as health information and education.

The Community shall complement the Member States' action in reducing drugs-related health damage, including information and prevention.

2. The Community shall encourage cooperation between the Member States in the areas referred to in this Article and, if necessary, lend support to their action.

Member States shall, in liaison with the Commission, coordinate among themselves their policies and programmes in the areas referred to in paragraph 1. The Commission may, in close contact with the Member States, take any useful initiative to promote such coordination.

3. The Community and the Member States shall foster cooperation with third countries and the competent international organizations in the sphere of public health.

4. The Council, acting in accordance with the procedure referred to in Article 251 and after consulting the Economic and Social Committee and the Committee of the Regions, shall contribute to the achievement of the objectives referred to in this article through adopting:

(a) measures setting high standards of quality and safety of organs and substances of human origin, blood and blood derivatives; these measures shall not prevent any Member State from maintaining or introducing more stringent protective measures;

(b) by way of derogation from Article 37, measures in the veterinary and phytosanitary fields which have as their direct objective the protection of public health;

(c) incentive measures designed to protect and improve human health, excluding any harmonization of the laws and regulations of the Member States.

The Council, acting by a qualified majority on a proposal from the Commission, may also adopt recommendations for the purposes set out in this article.

5. Community action in the field of public health shall fully respect the responsibilities of the Member States for the organization and delivery of health services and medical care. In particular, measures referred to in paragraph 4(a) shall not affect national provisions on the donation or medical use of organs and blood.

Treaty on the Functioning of the European Union (Lisbon, 2007)

From Title XIV – Public Health

Article 168 (ex Article 152 TEC)

1. A high level of human health protection shall be ensured in the definition and implementation of all Union policies and activities.

Union action, which shall complement national policies, shall be directed towards improving public health, preventing physical and mental illness and diseases, and obviating sources of danger to physical and mental health. Such action shall cover the fight against the major health scourges, by promoting research into their causes, their transmission and their prevention, as well as health information and education, and monitoring, early warning of and combating serious cross-border threats to health.

The Union shall complement the Member States' action in reducing drugs-related health damage, including information and prevention.

2. The Union shall encourage cooperation between the Member States in the areas referred to in this Article and, if necessary, lend support to their action. It shall in particular encourage cooperation between the Member States to improve the complementarity of their health services in cross-border areas.

Member States shall, in liaison with the Commission, coordinate among themselves their policies and programmes in the areas referred to in paragraph 1. The Commission may, in close contact with the Member States, take any useful initiative to promote such coordination, in particular initiatives aiming at the establishment of guidelines and indicators, the organization of exchange of best practice, and the preparation of the necessary elements for periodic monitoring and evaluation. The European Parliament shall be kept fully informed.

3. The Union and the Member States shall foster cooperation with third countries and the competent international organizations in the sphere of public health.

4. By way of derogation from Article 2(5) and Article 6(a) and in accordance with Article 4(2)(k) the European Parliament and the Council, acting in accordance with the ordinary legislative procedure and after consulting the Economic and Social Committee and the Committee of the Regions, shall contribute to the achievement of the objectives referred to in this Article through adopting in order to meet common safety concerns:

(a) measures setting high standards of quality and safety of organs and substances of human origin, blood and blood derivatives; these measures shall not prevent any Member State from maintaining or introducing more stringent protective measures;

(b) measures in the veterinary and phytosanitary fields which have as their direct objective the protection of public health;

(c) measures setting high standards of quality and safety for medicinal products and devices for medical use.

5. The European Parliament and the Council, acting in accordance with the ordinary legislative procedure and after consulting the Economic and Social Committee and the Committee of the Regions, may also adopt incentive measures designed to protect and improve human health and in particular to combat the major cross-border health scourges, measures concerning monitoring, early warning of and combating serious cross-border threats to health, and measures which have as their direct objective the protection of public health regarding tobacco and the abuse of

alcohol, excluding any harmonization of the laws and regulations of the Member States.

6. The Council, on a proposal from the Commission, may also adopt recommendations for the purposes set out in this Article.

7. Union action shall respect the responsibilities of the Member States for the definition of their health policy and for the organization and delivery of health services and medical care. The responsibilities of the Member States shall include the management of health services and medical care and the allocation of the resources assigned to them. The measures referred to in paragraph 4(a) shall not affect national provisions on the donation or medical use of organs and blood.

This background activity was overshadowed by what might be thought of as the EU's "foundational" health crisis, the BSE episode.[12] Bovine Spongiform Encephalopathy (BSE), nicknamed "mad cow" disease by the media, could if ingested by humans give them the alarming and fatal neurodegenerative variant Creutzfeldt-Jakob Disease (vCJD). Apart from the shocking images of dying cows and the terrifying implications for human victims, BSE had such impact because it revealed ways in which an established area of EU internal market activity, agriculture, was failing to regulate a rapidly changing food system. BSE was related to the sheep disease scrapie. It was being spread by agricultural techniques that turned rendered remains of dead animals into animal feed, thereby turning herbivorous food animals into not just carnivores but occasionally cannibals. Tracing infection proved extremely difficult due to limited and antiquated procedures for tracking animals or products. Member State relations deteriorated, with France putting an embargo on British meat in March 1996, other countries restricting blood donations by people who had eaten meat in the UK, and the UK press and government responding robustly to the insults being aimed at the national icon of British beef.[13] It seemed like a textbook example of an area in which European integration had outpaced the capacity, or political willingness, of the Member States to undertake coordinating activities at an intergovernmental level. Some sort of EU action would be necessary.

BSE struck in the midst of the preparations for what became known as the Treaty of Amsterdam, in which the health article was substantially expanded.

---

12 Of course, other crises have played a role in reshaping European and world health politics, such as the Thalidomide drugs scandal of the 1960s or the scandals to do with contaminated blood in France in the 1980s, which are still reverberating now: Steffen M (1999). "The nation's blood: Medicine, justice, and the State in France", in Feldman EA & Bayer R (eds.). Blood feuds: AIDS, blood, and the politics of medical disaster. New York: Oxford University Press, 95–126; Steffen M (2012). The Europeanization of public health: how does it work? The seminal role of the AIDS case. *Journal of Health Politics, Policy and Law*, 37(6):1057–89.

13 Ansell, C, Vogel D (eds.) (2006). *What's the Beef? The Contested Governance of European Food Safety* Cambridge, MA: MIT Press; Rogers B (2004). *Beef and Liberty*. Vintage.

The public health article, renamed Article 152 in the 1997 Amsterdam Treaty,[14] became longer, wordier and more ambitious, but it added only one concrete new EU power: a responsibility to regulate blood and blood products. Nonetheless, almost every key word remained noncoercive in EU law, from verbs such as "complement", "encourage" to "coordinate", to modifying clauses clarifying that the Member States' decision to coordinate is crucial, and EU institutions may support them, and finally to the last sentences, which make it clear that the public health article "shall fully respect" Member States' "organization and delivery of health services and medical care". At the same time as the development of the treaty base, European integration was proceeding apace in the area of food safety, on agricultural and other treaty bases (*see* chapter 3). Scandals involving dioxane-contaminated chicken in Belgium and the ongoing BSE problem kept the issue on the agenda, and the General Food Law was passed in 2002, harmonizing much practice and creating the European Food Safety Authority.

If the new public health treaty base authorized more public health ambition, there was still no agent in Brussels to promote public health. The Prodi Commission, however, created the Directorate-General for Public Health and Consumers, known awkwardly as DG SANCO, under the Irish Commissioner David Byrne (1999–2004). There were two basic reasons. The first was that the Prodi Commission took office in the wake of the resignation of the Santer Commission due to a corruption scandal, and the new College of Commissioners had an interest in showing a valuable face of the EU. The second, and most important, was that the BSE episode had not reinforced confidence in the old model of uniting regulatory and promotional functions in one organization, the directorate-general for agriculture. Moving health regulation away from its previous home in industry-promoting directorates such as agriculture was a way to strengthen public health and reduce bureaucratic and political incentives to downplay public health issues.

Once a policy arena exists in the EU, and once there is authorization to act for health, then the EU political system begins to reward policy entrepreneurs. The Health Strategy and Health Programme and the new Directorate-General for Health and Consumer Protection (DG SANCO at the time) anchored the new EU health policy arena, with a set of programmes, priorities, experts and advocates intersecting with the DG, the Commissioner and health ministers to define and act in the new EU policy arena.

Even as the EU's public health apparatus and ambition expanded, creating the first face of EU health policy as we know it, the second face made itself very visible to the health sectors of the EU in the way the EU's regulatory nature would lead us to expect: via a court case. The 1998 Kohll and Decker decisions

---

14 Which became effective in 1999.

by the European Court of Justice (ECJ, later renamed the Court of Justice of the European Union, CJEU) established the principle that the provision of health goods and services had to comply with internal market law, even when they were being financed through publicly funded healthcare systems, in this case Luxembourg's social insurance system. The cases immediately captured the attention of health interest groups, scholars and other courts. They started a long string of cases on patient mobility that made it clear that there was a European healthcare policy, that EU internal market law applied to healthcare activities in the eyes of the courts, and that the only way to constrain judicial application of internal market law was to start developing a European approach to healthcare services that would bring health objectives and expertise into the European system. It took some time for health advocates, ministers and ministries to recognize the paradoxical logic that the way to respond to an uninvited EU move into healthcare – the application of EU internal market law by courts – was to legislate at the EU level.

Patient mobility, a case of the EU legal system acting autonomously to expand the internal market, was a key reason for the birth of an EU policy sphere. It also gave rise to easily the largest literature on EU health policy, detailing the law and politics of this policy area. However inconsequential actual patient mobility in this particular legal framework may be, and inconsequential it has been, it was the policy area that made clear the Europeanization of healthcare policy and politics, as well as its limits.[15] At the end was the Directive on Cross-Border Patient Mobility, discussed in section 4.3.1. While formally it was an internal market policy, its passage at least established that healthcare services are not like any other services and health stakeholders were strong enough to establish this.[16]

---

15 Brooks E (2012). Crossing Borders: A Critical Review of the Role of the European Court of Justice in EU Health Policy. *Health Policy*, 105:33–7; Obermaier AJ (2009). *The End of Territoriality? The Impact of ECJ Rulings on British, German and French Social Policy.* Aldershot: Ashgate; McKee M, Mossialos E, Baeten R (eds.) (2002). *The Impact of EU Law on Health Care Systems.* Brussels: Peter Lang; McKee M, Mossialos E, Baeten R (eds.) (2002). *EU Law and the Social Character of Health Care.* Brussels: Peter Lang; Busse R, Wismar M, Berman PC (eds.) (2002). *The European Union and Health Services: The Impact of the Single European Market on Member States.* Amsterdam: IOS/European Health Management Association; Wasserfallen F (2010). The Judiciary as Legislator? How the European Court of Justice Shapes Policy-Making in the European Union. *Journal of European Public Policy*, 17:1128–46; Martinsen DS (2005). Towards an Internal Health Market With the European Court. *West European Politics*, 28:1035–56; Greer SL (2006). Uninvited Europeanization: Neofunctionalism and the EU in Health Policy. *Journal of European Public Policy*, 13:134–52; Lamping W, Steffen M (2009). European Union and Health Policy: The "chaordic" Dynamics of Integration. *Social Science Quarterly*, 90:1361–79; Martinsen DS (2015). *An ever more powerful court?: The political constraints of legal integration in the European Union.* Oxford: Oxford University Press.

16 Greer SL (2008). Choosing Paths in European Union Health Policy: A Political Analysis of a Critical Juncture. *Journal of European Social Policy*, 18:219–31; Greer SL (2009). "The Changing World of European Health Lobbies", in Coen D & Richardson JJ (eds.). *Lobbying in the European Union.* Oxford: Oxford University Press; Greer SL (2013). Avoiding Another Directive: The Unstable Politics of European Union Cross-Border Health Care Law. *Health Economics, Policy and Law*, 8(4):415–21.

EU public health policy, meanwhile, took its next steps forward with strong tobacco control legislation (3.1.1.) and the institutionalization of its role in communicable disease control. Severe Acute Respiratory Syndrome (SARS) had essentially no impact on European public health but it shook policy-makers worldwide and created a new interest in communicable disease control. Bio-terrorism in the United States in 2001 using weaponized anthrax was also a worrisome precedent, and new pandemic influenzas were looming as an increasingly important threat. Given that for various reasons public health was becoming increasingly visible and important as a political agenda item in its own right around Europe, including in France, Germany and the UK, the result was support for a strong EU role in communicable disease control. Using Article 168, the EU institutions created the European Centre for Disease Control and Prevention, an EU agency tasked with rationalizing, strengthening and coordinating EU and Member State activities for health, with a special initial focus on surveillance, science, and preparing for and assisting Member States with responses to new health threats.

EU health policy was not a priority of the 2014–2019 Juncker Commission, which promised to be "big on the big things and small on the small things",[17] and gave a strong impression that health was a "small thing". In the aftermath of the UK's 2016 Brexit vote, the Commission even produced a strategy paper with one of the five options being an EU that did nothing on or for health.[18] Despite this broad trend, EU health policy has not gone away since the previous (2014) edition of this book. DG SANTE has spearheaded a number of important policies for health (*see* chapter 3) and over the last five years steadily incorporated health goals into internal market (chapter 4) and fiscal governance policies (chapter 5). The Juncker Commission priorities allowed Commissioner Andriukaitis to place health and food safety priorities in other policy areas and there have also been major advances in SDG3 (Box 2.6). Moreover, the Commissioner went beyond his limited mission letter (Appendix IV), in introducing a range of initiatives and legislative changes such as in tobacco control and general food legislation.

For most of the continent the five years of the Juncker Commission have been focused on economic issues, including battles about austerity and the nature and speed of the economic recovery, on the rule of law, and on arguments about migration. The UK, though, created a special set of problems with its Brexit vote in 2016. The effects of Brexit on the health and health system of the UK will be very serious. The potential impact on health of the UK leaving the European Union illustrates the range of ways in which the EU has an impact on health policy. Table 1.1 illustrates this, breaking down the range of potential impacts

---

17 A statement that Jean-Claude Juncker made a number of times in key speeches, e.g. his 2018 State of the Union speech. Available at: http://europa.eu/rapid/press-release_SPEECH-18-5808_en.htm.

18 European Commission (2017). *White Paper on the Future of Europe: Five Scenarios.*

from Brexit by rows according to the health system building blocks of the World Health Organization.[19] The columns describe four possible outcomes: (1) a "No Deal" Brexit under which the UK leaves the EU without any formal agreement on the terms of withdrawal; (2) the Withdrawal Agreement, as negotiated between the UK and EU and awaiting (possible) formal agreement, which provides a transition period until the end of December 2020; (3) if the Northern Ireland Protocol's 'Backstop' comes into effect after the end of that period; and (4) the Political Declaration on the Future Relationship between the UK and the EU. As this shows, all of these scenarios for Brexit have negative consequences for the UK's NHS across a wide range of areas. Moreover, the largest impact may come from none of these direct areas, but from Brexit's impact on the wider UK economy and thus on the ability of the UK to finance its health service.

The effects on the policies and health of the rest of the EU are less clear. The departure of the UK unequivocally reduces the size of the EU population, economy and budget, with effects on its position in world affairs. But internally, it also weakens the liberal block in the EU that has promoted deregulation through the internal market.[20] The EU after Brexit will not just have the ongoing policy agenda of managing relations with the UK,[21] or rebuilding policy expertise in areas where it depended on the UK. It will also have a new politics in which liberalization is less politically powerful and France is relatively empowered. That will be a new experience for those familiar with the EU since UK accession in 1973.

1.4 Three dynamics of EU health policy

What does this history tell us about the evolution of European Union health policies? Broadly, there are three themes. The first is that integration begets integration.[22] Integration of agricultural markets led to pressure for integration of regulatory frameworks after BSE struck. Integration of internal market law led to its application to healthcare services, which led to health stakeholders

---

19 Fahy N et al. (2019). How will Brexit affect health services in the UK? An updated evaluation. *The Lancet*, 393(10174):949–58. Available at: https://doi.org/10.1016/S0140-6736(19)30425-8.

20 Greer SL, Laible J (eds.)(2020). *The European Union After Brexit*. Manchester University Press.

21 At the time of writing (summer 2019), the health dimensions of Brexit's impact on the EU cannot be known in detail since everything from a "hard Brexit", with almost every legal relationship with the UK undone, to the UK remaining, is possible. Many of the practical issues are to do with the UK's only land border, with the Republic of Ireland. Valuable background reading that captures many of the underlying constraints on any discussion of that topic is: De Mars S et al. (2018). *Bordering two unions: Northern Ireland and Brexit*. Bristol: Policy Press.

22 Greer SL (2006). Uninvited Europeanization: Neofunctionalism and the EU in Health Policy. *Journal of European Public Policy*, 13:134–52.

Table 1.1 *Impact of four different Brexit scenarios*

		No Deal Brexit	Transition (the WA)	Backstop (NI Protocol)	Future relationship
Workforce	Recruitment and retention of EU nationals in the NHS	No provisions facilitating recruitment and retention of NHS workers.	Legal framework continues with some changes, retention and recruitment continues. Uncertainty over administrative arrangements.	The Backstop does not include protections for residency of EU/EEA nationals. Irish nationals in the UK do not need new status; all other EEA nationals do.	No provisions facilitating recruitment and retention of NHS workers.
	Mutual recognition of professional qualifications	Theoretical potential to improve standards likely to be hampered in practice by recruitment needs. Mutual recognition and protections it gives stops immediately, and will limit information exchange about health professionals moving across Europe.	The existing provisions for mutual recognition of professional qualifications and the related alert mechanisms will continue.	Theoretical potential to improve standards likely to be hampered in practice by recruitment needs. No provisions for mutual recognition beyond end of transitional period.	Declaration indicates weak ambition for arrangements on mutual recognition of professional qualifications; but this is already less ambitious than the Canada-EU Free Trade Agreement, which has not yet led to any substantive cooperation.
	Employment rights for health workers	No protection other than in domestic law of existing rights.	Legal framework continues.	Legal framework continues under some 'level playing field' rules in employment law. Nationality is not a forbidden ground of discrimination under these laws.	Typically FTAs like CETA do not involve enforceable employment rights provisions.

continued overleaf >

Grey = broadly unchanged; Green = positive; Pale Red = moderate negative; Red = major negative

establishing a presence in Brussels and seeking to create legislation that better suited the health sector.[23]

The second follows logically: integration exists and proceeds regardless of whether it is wanted, but what it means and how much it matters can vary and is responsive to the preferences of Member States and health stakeholders. The debate about

---

23   Vollaard H (2017). Patient mobility, changing territoriality and scale in the EU's internal market. *Comparative European Politics*, 15(3):435–58; Greer SL (2006). Uninvited Europeanization: Neofunctionalism and the EU in Health Policy. *Journal of European Public Policy*, 13:134–52.

Table 1.1 *Impact of four different Brexit scenarios [continued]*

		No Deal Brexit	Transition (the WA)	Backstop (NI Protocol)	Future relationship
Financing	Reciprocal healthcare arrange-ments	No rights in place as legal framework ceases immediately.	Existing mechanism for coordination of social security continues. May be practical registration issues.	No provision for continued reciprocal arrangements for social security under the Northern Ireland Protocol.	Potential for some weaker form of reciprocal healthcare coordination than currently, but linked to future free movement between the UK and the EU.
	Capital financing for the NHS	Access to EIB stopped and capital financing generally undermined.	Legal framework continues for existing EIB financed projects but no new financing from the EIB.	Access to EIB stopped and capital financing generally undermined.	Potential to participate in and receive funding from the EIB; likely lower level of capital financing than currently.
	Indirect impact on NHS financing	Severe effect on wider economy and thus NHS financing.	Some effect on wider economy and thus NHS financing.	Some effect on wider economy and thus NHS financing.	Some effect on wider economy and thus NHS financing.
Medical products, vaccines and technol-ogy	Pharmaceu-ticals	Absence of legal framework for imports/exports drastically affects supply chains. Major disruption expected.	Continued application of EU law to circulation of medicinal products. For regulation and licensing, the UK becomes a rule-taker. Loss of global influence through role in European Medicines Agency.	Continued application of EU law to circulation of medicinal products. Special arrangements for medicines manufactured in Northern Ireland. For regulation and licensing, the UK would not be able to license products for the EU.	Potential for some weaker cooperation with EU on licensing and regulation of medicines than currently.
	Other medical products	Major concerns about timely access to radioisotopes.	Continuity of supply secured.	As for pharmaceuticals.	As for pharmaceuticals.

continued overleaf

Grey = broadly unchanged; Green = positive; Pale Red = moderate negative; Red = major negative

EU policy on healthcare services regulation was about what kind of regulatory framework it would be, what it would try to do, what policy instruments it would use, which parts of the Council and Commission would manage it, what the role of the courts would be, and what its priorities would be – in other words, almost everything. The fact that an EU health policy exists is less important than what is done with it and to whom it matters. Sometimes there is a debate about whether EU policies in an area should be viewed as a policy area, as with debates about

Table 1.1   *Impact of four different Brexit scenarios [continued]*

		No Deal Brexit	Transition (the WA)	Backstop (NI Protocol)	Future relationship
Information		Absence of legal framework means end of information collaboration based on EU law.	Current legal framework continues; current information exchange activities continue.	Access only to information systems related to circulation of goods (ie: pharmaceuticals, medical devices) and substances of human origin (eg: blood). Access to other health-related information systems ends.	No specific cooperation on health information envisaged.
Service delivery	Working Time legislation	Regulation of working time and other conditions of work formally returns to the UK, but scope to change in practice is limited.	Legal framework continues.	Legal framework continues under level playing field rules in NI Protocol.	Regulation of working time and other conditions of work formally returns to the UK, but scope to change in practice is limited.
	Cross-border care	No framework for cross-border care to cope with long waiting times and administration/ offset between UK and EU countries.	Legal framework continues.	Not covered, except for island of Ireland implicitly and as part of the Co-operation and Working Together (CAWT) to promote peace and reconciliation.	Cross-border health services not envisaged as part of the future relationship.
Leadership and govern-ance	Public health	The government has offered reassurances to maintain EU standards but refused to enshrine them in legislation. Absence of EU law means that upholding public health standards in future depends on the political will of the government of the day.	Legal framework continues but the UK is outside EU institutional structures so loss of role in e.g. ECDC.	Government reassurances to maintain EU standards, but scope to improve public health standards is contingent on political will. Limited or no participation in decisions by e.g. ECDC.	Impact of EU rules dependent on depth of partnership. Limited or no participation in decisions by e.g. ECDC.
		Existing protections can be removed by executive action.	No mention in WA.	Existing protections can be removed by executive action.	Continued collaboration on public health at global level.

continued overleaf >

Grey = broadly unchanged; Green = positive; Pale Red = moderate negative; Red = major negative

Table 1.1 *Impact of four different Brexit scenarios [continued]*

		No Deal Brexit	Transition (the WA)	Backstop (NI Protocol)	Future relationship
Leadership and govern-ance (continued)	Trade and competition	NHS (England) no longer operates in perceived shadow of EU competition and public procurement law provisions which are felt to drive inefficient behaviours in the context of the NHS.	Legal framework continues but the UK is outside EU institutional structures so loss of role.	Legal framework continues under NIP level playing field rules.	Impact of EU rules dependent on depth of partnership.
		Outside EU trade structures, the UK's global influence over health in trade deals is reduced (further). Some existing protections could be removed by executive action.			
	Research	Collaborations and funding from EU ended. No access to Clinical Trials Reg's portal. Loss of global influence.	Collaborations and funding, plus legal framework, continue until the end of 2020.	Product access, but otherwise collaborations and funding from EU ended. Loss of global influence.	Continued participation in research envisaged, but on worse terms for the UK. Loss of global leadership and influence.
	Scrutiny and stakeholder engage-ment	Volume of new legislation already limiting scrutiny and engagement, will continue.	Volume of new legislation and executive powers under EU (W) Act limits scrutiny and engagement.	Volume of new legislation and executive powers under EU (W) Act, plus new trade agreements, limits scrutiny and engagement.	Volume of new legislation and executive powers under EU (W) Act, plus new trade agreements, limits scrutiny and engagement.

Grey = broadly unchanged; Green = positive; Pale Red = moderate negative; Red = major negative

the presence of a European health law,[24] or the struggles over whether the many EU actions that affect the consumption and effect of alcohol or food should be viewed as a coherent policy area that should take health seriously (chapter 3).

The third is that crises and shocks get attention. It is a staple of public health history that crises provoke action and public health initiatives arise after outbreaks.

---

24 Hervey TK, McHale JV (2015). *European Union health law*. Cambridge: Cambridge University Press.

The big steps in EU public health policy do seem to follow threats, in particular with BSE and the creation of the health DG and then the increased number of communicable disease crises and the creation of the ECDC. Crises are what political scientists call "focusing events" – they focus attention on the issue. Public health crises put public health on the agenda, bringing seemingly technical microbiology and epidemiology out of the shadows into the centre of public attention, and are an opportunity for entrepreneurs to push forth public health initiatives that were being neglected.

1.5   The emergence of a variable EU health policy arena

We have spoken so far mostly about the areas in which the EU acts in traditional and core areas of health policy: healthcare and public health. But there are four parts of the Treaty on the Functioning of the European Union (TFEU) that explicitly make better health a European Union goal, as discussed in chapter 2. Alongside the public health Article 168, there are articles about the environment (191), labour in the Social Policy chapter (153, 156) and consumer protection (169) that specify health as an objective. This is a field in which the EU already does much for health – some of its individual environmental policies, in particular, might have prevented more avoidable deaths than all the policies it has made in the name of health and healthcare. Finally, Article 9 calls for all EU activity to "take into account" a "high level of protection of human health".

In other words, the treaties lay out areas where there is clear authorization to act with health as an objective, and it is hard to argue that health is an illegitimate or unusual goal in environmental, labour and consumer protection. These are not just areas where the EU's health effects are already visible and often positive; they are areas where there is authorization in the treaties for more, and more coordinated, efforts to improve health.

Beyond those treaty articles, the three faces of the EU health policy look upon many of the social determinants of health, from regulating food labelling to subsidizing agriculture, to encouraging raising pension ages, to making trade agreements, to building infrastructure that might or might not encourage walking and cycling.[25] Within Member States, it has long been recognized that the healthcare system is only one contributor to health. The EU has policy levers

---

25 Consider one example of European integration with health consequences: the European Road Safety Observatory, born of EU-funded research projects but now maintained by the Commission's transport DG, making its contribution to Europe's world-leading road safety: *see* https://ec.europa.eu/transport/road_safety/specialist/erso_en. Or, still in the field of transport, consider EU vehicle safety rules made as part of the single internal market. EU legislation frames the safety of vehicles in terms of deaths in and outside the vehicle, while US law defines safety purely in terms of the effects of crashes on people *inside* the vehicle. This basic legal framework means there are tens of thousands of people alive in Europe who, in the United States, would probably be dead.

over many of the most powerful determinants of health and in some areas such as agriculture or trade is one of the most powerful actors in Europe or the world. To promote health is to understand and seek to use this EU leverage.

1.6   Health, convergence and the EU

The European Union has 28 Member States (27 after the expected departure of the UK) and around 512 million people (about 446 million without the UK), making it one of the world's largest political units compared to the US (327 million), China (1 386 million), India (1 399 million) and Japan (126 million). It is also extremely diverse – economically, culturally, politically and in health terms. For understanding the background of health policy in particular, it is worth remembering both the different economic and health outcomes and the extent of convergence. In particular, it is worth noting the extent to which convergence between different Member States is not clearly continuing, whether in GDP (which was in France 1.160 trillion (current) US dollars in 1995, 2.196 trillion in 2005 and 2.438 trillion in 2015; in Spain 612.94 billion (current) US dollars in 1995, 1.157 trillion in 2005 and 1.199 trillion in 2015; and in Greece 136.878 billion (current) US dollars in 1995, 247.783 billion in 2005 and 196.591 billion in 2015)[26] or life expectancy at birth (which was in France 77.751 years in 1995, 80.163 in 2005 and 82.322 in 2015; in Spain 77.981 years in 1995, 80.171 in 2005 and 82.832 in 2015; and in Greece 77.585 years in 1995, 79.239 in 2005 and 81.037 in 2015).[27] Perhaps unsurprisingly, the percentage of GDP spent on health varies substantially (in France, 10.18% of GDP in 2005 and 11.501% in 2015; in Spain 7.676% in 2005 and 9.12% in 2015; and in Greece 8.997% in 2005 and 8.194% in 2015).[28] More surprising perhaps is the variation in healthy life years relative to life expectancy, which among other things shows and predicts the extent to which older people are faring well (average healthy life years at birth were, for Swedish men, 67 years in 2010 and 72 years in 2016; for Danish men, 60 years in 2010 and 62 years in 2016; and for Slovakian men, 52 years in 2010 and 57 in 2016).[29]

In other words, convergence within the EU is neither inevitable nor necessarily proceeding under the current policy regime. Fig. 1.1 shows trends in convergence in GDP per capita since 1995, showing that overall economic convergence is

---

26 World Bank Data. "GDP (current US$)". Available at: https://data.worldbank.org/indicator/NY.GDP. MKTP.CD?locations=FR-ES-GR.

27 World Bank Data. "Life expectancy at birth, total (years)". Available at: https://data.worldbank.org/ indicator/SP.DYN.LE00.IN?locations=FR-ES-GR.

28 World Bank Data. "Current health expenditure (% of GDP)". Available at: https://data.worldbank.org/ indicator/SH.XPD.CHEX.GD.ZS?locations=FR-ES-GR.

29 Eurostat. "Healthy life years at birth, male, 2010 and 2016". Available at: https://ec.europa.eu/eurostat/ statistics-explained/index.php?title=File:Healthy_life_years_at_birth,_males,_2010_and_2016_(years)_ YB17.png.

Box 1.5   *Well-being*

The treaties state the overall aim of the EU as being "to promote peace, its values and the well-being of its peoples" (emphasis added).[a] Although not directly a reference to health, this of course echoes both the World Health Organization's definition of health ("Health is a state of complete physical, mental and social well-being and not merely the absence of disease or infirmity")[b] and the objectives for improving well-being set by the WHO's European "Health 2020" strategy.[c]

The treaty aim does not have any specific powers attached to it – rather, all the powers in the treaties are intended to help to achieve this overall aim. There has been some specific work related to this, however, centered on the idea of developing broader measures of progress in European countries than the traditional summary of GDP,[d] within which health is one of the main dimensions. This has been followed by a range of reports and publications by the EU, by Member States and by other international bodies.[e]

It has received a push in 2019. The Finnish Presidency of the Council released draft conclusions (for the September EPSCO meeting[f]) on the economy of well-being as a "policy orientation and governance approach" that "brings into focus the *raison d'être* of the EU as enshrined in the treaties and in the Charter of Fundamental Rights of the European Union". An economy of well-being, it continues, entails cross-sectoral collaborations (noting Health in All Policies) and includes access to healthcare, "promotion of health and preventative measures" and "occupational health and safety".

However, although there is by now an extensive range of reports and evidence highlighting the relevance of these broader concepts of development and well-being and the importance of health as one of the key issues, it is not clear that this evidence has yet brought about any substantive changes in policy-making. With the agreement of the Sustainable Development Goals (SDGs) in 2015, it may be that in practice the SDGs and their monitoring will prove to be the primary focus for efforts to take a broader perspective on development, rather than the concept of well-being.

[a]   Treaty on the European Union, Article 3.

[b]   Preamble to the Constitution of the WHO as adopted by the International Health Conference, New York, 19–22 June 1946, signed on 22 July 1946 by the representatives of 61 States (Official Records of the World Health Organization, no. 2, p. 100) and entered into force on 7 April 1948.

[c]   WHO Regional Office for Europe (2013). *The European health report 2012: charting the way to well-being and Health 2020: a European policy framework and strategy for the 21st century.* Copenhagen: WHO Regional Office for Europe.

[d]   European Commission (2009). *Communication: GDP and beyond – measuring progress in a changing world (COM(2009)433).* Brussels: European Commission.

[e]   *See* http://ec.europa.eu/environment/beyond_gdp/index_en.html for more information.

[f]   Council of the European Union (21 June 2019). The Economy of Well-Being. Executive Summary of the OECD Background Paper on "Creating opportunities for people's well-being and economic growth". Brussels. Available at: https://data.consilium.europa.eu/doc/document/ST-10414-2019-INIT/en/pdf.

Fig. 1.1 *GDP per capita, PPP (current international $)*

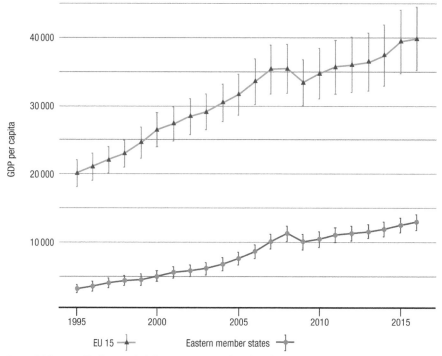

Source: Makszin K (forthcoming). "The East-West Divide: Obstacles to European Integration" in Greer SL and Laible J (eds.), *The European Union after Brexit*. Manchester: Manchester University Press.

not the main story of the twenty-first century EU. Trends in health show a similar pattern.

1.7 Conclusion

In the EU, having a legal basis provides the crucial authorization for policy entrepreneurship,[30] but the public health legal basis is so weak as to impede even discussion of possible fruitful EU health policy.

To sharpen the point, the EU treaties prevent much activity grounded in the public health article, but that manifestly does not mean that the EU lacks health policy. Instead, it means that the EU's health policies are made under other guises, as part of efforts to promote and regulate the internal market, to ensure the protection of workers, consumers and the environment, to invest in poorer regions or to monitor the fiscal decisions of its Member States. There are powerful tools there, but in each case they legally, politically and practically

---

30 Page EC (2012). "The European Commission Bureaucracy: Handling Sovereignty Through the Back and Front Doors", in Hayward J & Wurzel R (eds.). *European Disunion: Between Sovereignty and Solidarity*. Basingstoke: Palgrave Macmillan.

belong to another sector. There can be and is an EU policy on acceptable rules for developing baskets of covered healthcare services, but it cannot be made with health as its declared primary goal, just as there are EU recommendations, some very specific and backed by the threat of fines, to Member States about how to operate their health systems, but they cannot primarily be made with health, as against fiscal sustainability, as their goal.

If Article 9's commitment that the EU shall always take into account "protection of human health" is to carry any weight, the solution cannot be limited to the weak public health treaty article; it will be in understanding and finding ways to gain leverage over multiple powerful and promising elements of EU policy, from the European Semester to medical devices regulation.

The last five years have shown what can be done within the limits of Article 168 and an overall EU political agenda that was focused elsewhere. Health policies we discuss range from the State of Health in the EU reports to tobacco control and European Reference Networks, and the Commission, particularly DG SANTE, has taken action in crucial areas such as healthy lifestyles, vaccination and antimicrobial resistance. Combined with action across the EU's many other policies, where health has gained prominence over the term of the Juncker Commission, the result has shaped health outcomes and shows how powerful, and inescapable, EU health policy can be. Comparing the very minimal goals of the 2014 Mandate letter to Commissioner Andriukitis with the results we describe in this book makes the point: health can be put on the EU agenda and advanced as a goal even against political headwinds.

Chapter 2

The European Union: institutions, processes and powers

This chapter introduces the EU institutions and a few key points for the analysis and interpretation of EU health policy. For health policy-makers, the first key point is that EU regulation and law are powerful tools to promote health, but those tools are often organized – bureaucratically, politically and legally –under some other title such as environmental or social policy. Neither healthcare nor health outcomes in the EU can be understood without considering the full range of legal bases and tools the EU can use.

The second key point is that the EU's impact on healthcare has been mostly indirect or limited, although one of the consequences of the 2008 financial crisis has been to increase its direct influence. The limited action on health and healthcare comes about for deep legal and political reasons. Despite consensus on the importance of good and generally egalitarian health as one of Europe's most distinctive features,[1] in successive treaty revisions national governments have preferred to keep health issues primarily at national level and so have provided only limited powers for EU action in pursuit of health. However, health is affected by many wider social and environmental factors on which the EU has its own impact, and health systems form one of the largest sectors of the European economy.[2] In 2018 health spending accounted for nearly 10% of GDP in the EU, with France and Germany allocating more than 11% of their GDP to health spending.[3]

As a result, health and health systems are most affected at EU level by policies born in other sectors, particularly those affecting the determinants of health (such as environmental policy), the integration of the internal market (through issues such as cross-border healthcare or professional mobility) and health regulation (as with regulations on labour and pharmaceuticals). Reflecting the origins of the

---

1   Council of the European Union (2006). Council conclusions on common values and principles in European health systems. *Official Journal*, C146:1–4.
2   OECD (2012). *Health at a glance: Europe 2012*. Paris: Organisation for Economic Co-operation and Development.
3   OECD (2018). *Health at a glance: Europe 2018 – State of health in the EU cycle*. Joint publication of the OECD and the European Commission. Paris: Organisation for Economic Co-operation and Development.

EU, these are policy areas where the EU is built to produce market integration, economic growth and development through the extension of single market law.[4]

Despite this asymmetry in the EU's approach towards health, the EU does have a substantial range of policies that affect health, and an increasing number of initiatives that try to promote health or counteract potentially unhelpful effects of other policies on health.

2.1 European political institutions

The EU has three core institutions: an executive (the European Commission), two legislative bodies (the European Parliament, with members (MEPs) elected by direct vote in each Member State, and the Council of Ministers, comprising national ministers from each Member State), and a Court of Justice.

2.1.1 The European Commission

The executive body of the EU is the European Commission, which is made up of individual commissioners, one from each Member State and appointed by agreement between the Parliament and the Council. In addition to their personal office (or cabinet), these commissioners are supported by directorates-general (DGs), akin to ministries; each has a name and a shorthand name usually presented in capital letters.[5] Commission Vice-Presidents chosen from among the Commissioners oversee groups of individual Commissioners on broad topics and are important figures.

In July 2019 the European Council nominated Ursula von der Leyen to succeed Juncker, and she was approved as Commission President that month. She won the support of 383 MEPs, nine votes more than required to secure an absolute majority in a secret ballot.

The most obvious actor for health and health systems up to September 2019 is the DG for Health, known from its acronym in French as DG SANTE (and known, until 2014, when it lost consumer protection, as the Directorate-General for Health and Consumers, or DG SANCO). Twenty years old in 2019, it is responsible for EU policies in public health and food safety, which include cross-border healthcare and tobacco control, as well as pharmaceuticals, State of Health in the EU, and medical devices (which was just moved over from the reputedly more pro-industry DG Enterprise, now DG Internal Market,

---

4   European Commission (2010). *Europe 2020: a strategy for smart, sustainable and inclusive growth.* Luxembourg: Publications Office of the European Union.
5   For a complete list, *see* European Commission (2019). *Departments (Directorates-General) and Executive Agencies.* Brussels: European Commission. Available at: https://ec.europa.eu/info/departments_en, accessed 30 April 2019.

Industry, Entrepreneurship and SMEs, aka DG GROW).[6] Other DGs have more specialized but consequential roles to play for health systems. Each of the policy areas that lead to their involvement will be discussed in this book:

DG Research and Innovation is in charge of the substantial EU research budget, which often finances biomedical and health-related research;

DG Regional and Urban Policy is responsible for managing structural funds, the EU's regional development aid system, which is important to the finances of recipient regions and finances substantial health infrastructure;

DG Competition is responsible for the development and application of competition law and state aids, which has touched on the organization of healthcare in a variety of cases;

DG Communications Networks, Content and Technology is a major funder and policy-maker in health information technology and e-health;

DG Internal Market, Industry, Entrepreneurship and SMEs (small businesses) is the guardian of the internal market law and its enforcement, which made it a major part of the story of cross-border patient mobility;

DG Employment, Social Affairs and Inclusion has a major role in EU social policy; in addition to its responsibility for health and safety, it touches on health via its broad social policy proposals, its administration of the European Social Fund and its administration of social security coordination, which includes much cross-border healthcare;

DG Eurostat is the statistical office of the EU, responsible for publishing Europe-wide statistics and indicators that enable comparisons between countries and regions. DG Eurostat frequently publishes health policy indicators; and

DG Trade negotiates for the EU in its international trade dealings, including with the World Trade Organization and in bilateral trade agreements.

Stella Kyriakides was nominated as Commissioner-designate for Health on 10 September, 2019. A clinical psychologist by training, Kyriakides served prior to her nomination in Cyprus' House of Representatives. She worked on health and social policy issues, including breast cancer prevention. According to a mission letter sent to Kyriakides by President-elect Von der Leyen on 10 September,

---

6   See Appendices IV and V which reproduce contents of the Mission Letters spelling out the priorities that new Commission Presidents set for Commissioners Andriukaitis and Kyriakides.

2019, the new Commissioner for health will be responsible for "promoting and protecting public health" and ensuring "food safety and animal and plant health".[7]

As part of her mission letter, Kyriakides is asked to help ensure that the European Union has a steady supply of affordable medicines and will be responsible for the effective implementation of the new framework on medical devices adopted in 2017. Special attention will be given to health technologies and e-health, through the creation of a European Health Data Space that will promote health-data exchange and support research on new preventive initiatives.[8] The new Commissioner will also focus on the implementation of the European One Health Action Plan against Antimicrobial Resistance. Finally, the mission letter mentions that all Commissioners will be asked to contribute to the implementation of the Sustainable Development Goals.

DG Health (DG SANTE) will thus undergo several structural changes. Medical devices regulation will move back from DG GROW to DG SANTE.[9] Von der Leyen has also put together a College that is responsible for implementing the "Political Guidelines for the next European Commission" that she presented on 6 July, 2019. The new College will have eight Vice-Presidents, Commmissioner Kyriakides' mission letter directs her to work with the Vice-President for the European Green Deal, Frans Timmermans, on food safety and animal and plant health, and with the Vice-President for Protecting Our European Way of Life, Margaritis Schinas, on public health.[10]

Health systems, of course, are not the whole of health policy, and a number of DGs that are not widely seen as part of the health sector play an important role in shaping the health of Europeans. A few that are particularly powerful within the EU and affect health in Europe are DG Agriculture and Rural Development, which administers and helps to shape EU food and agriculture policy; and DG Environment, which works on environmental protection, where the EU has extensive powers that have afforded Europeans a comparatively high level of protection from myriad environmental threats to health. For those outside the EU, its important development, crisis response and, in some cases, neighbourhood policies, all of which influence global health, are the responsibility of DG International Cooperation and Development, DG European Civil Protection and Humanitarian Aid Operations, and DG European Neighbourhood Policy and Enlargement Negotiations, depending on the country and issue concerned.

---

7   European Commission. Ursula von der Leyen, President-elect of the European Commission. "Mission Letter. Stella Kyriakides". Brussels, 10 September, 2019. The text of the letter is reproduced as Appendix V.
8   Idem.
9   European Commission. 2019-2024. "Allocations of Portefolios and Supporting Services". 10 September 2019.
10   European Commission. "The von der Leyen Commission: for a Union that strives for more". Press Release. Brussels, 10 September 2019.

Box 2.1   *Commission proposal development*

The European Commission is responsible for planning, preparing and proposing new European legislation. In an attempt to increase transparency and policy coherence, the Barroso Commission introduced a requirement in policy-making that includes publishing the intention to present a proposal at the earliest stage on a publicly accessible road map.* Roadmaps seek to describe the problem to be tackled and the objectives to be met by the new legislation. They also explain why EU legislation is needed and describe the main features of the consultation strategy. Legislative and other important proposals should be introduced by a consultative document, followed by a public consultation and a Commission impact assessment focusing on economic, environmental and social aspects (including impact on public health and health systems under the social pillar). Any important proposal needs to pass the impact assessment board, composed of directors from the coordinating DGs and the economic, environmental and social DGs, before it can be agreed internally. In this case, the roadmap is replaced by an inception impact assessment, which goes into greater detail.

* European Commission (2013). *2013 roadmaps.* Luxembourg: Publications Office of the European Union. Available at: http://ec.europa.eu/governance/impact/planned_ia/roadmaps_2013_en.htm#SANCO, accessed 4 July 2014.

The Commission acts highly collectively in its decision-making and has strong internal mechanisms supporting the College of Commissioners to ensure that collective approach, with any decision by the Commission subject to multiple levels of internal consultation – between DGs (referred to as interservice consultation), between the cabinets of the commissioners and through collective consideration by the College of Commissioners themselves. The European Commission is supported by the Secretariat-General, which is responsible for coordinating the work across the entire Commission to make sure that all initiatives are aligned with the political priorities of the President, and for steering these new policies through the other EU institutions.

By the standards of the national government of a large country such as the United Kingdom or France, the Commission is a relatively small body (although at 32 399 staff[11] – as of April 2019 – it is still substantial). That small size is misleading, since the Commission is almost entirely dedicated to policy-making. It can influence most aspects of life in Europe with fewer employees than many regional governments because it does not have employees who sweep streets or drive buses. The Member States do the implementation and much of the actual detailed policy formulation, in a system of outsourcing that makes the EU a remarkably efficient policy-making mechanism.[12] The Commission also has

---

11   European Commission (2019). *Human resources key figures card: staff members.* Luxembourg: Publications Office of the European Union.

12   Page EC (2001). "The European Union and the bureaucratic mode of production", in Menon A (ed.). *From the nation state to Europe: essays in honour of Jack Hayward.* Oxford: Oxford University Press.

what is termed the "right of initiative". EU legislation, although decided by the Council and Parliament, can only begin with a Commission proposal, which gives the Commission enormous influence in shaping the detailed content of a proposal (though given that both Councils and the Parliament can and do request the Commission to bring forward particular proposals, this is less of a restriction than it might seem).

The Commission does not just act through legislative proposals, of course; it typically announces its priorities and approaches to its responsibilities in *Communications*, as well as using tools such as financing. *Communications* are documents that are politically and technically vetted within the Commission, usually with an eye on the broader context. Even old *Communications* from previous Commission leadership will often still be taken as the authorization for certain policies or ways of thinking. The Commission has the power to take its own direct *Decisions* in some areas, in particular for competition rulings.

Since April 2012, by means of the European Citizens' Initiative (ECI) introduced by the Lisbon Treaty, EU citizens may call on the Commission to make proposals. Two out of the four initiatives[13] that have successfully reached the required number of statements of support since 2012 deal with health issues. In the first ECI made in 2012,[14] EU citizens asked the Commission to propose legislation implementing a human right to water and sanitation, as recognized by the United Nations. The Commission committed in 2013[15] to take a series of actions reinforcing implementation of EU water quality legislation.

More recently, in January 2017, EU citizens also called on the Commission to propose to Member States a ban on glyphosate and to reform the EU pesticide approval procedure and set EU-wide mandatory reduction targets for pesticide use.[16] Although the Commission concluded in December 2017[17] that there were "neither scientific nor legal grounds to justify a ban of glyphosate". DG SANTE responded quickly. A proposal on transparency and sustainability of the EU risk assessment in the food chain was adopted by the Commission in April 2018[18] in response to the second aim of the initiative (to "ensure that the scientific

---

13 A list of successful "European Citizens' Initiatives" can be found here: http://ec.europa.eu/citizens-initiative/public/initiatives/successful.

14 European Commission (2012). The European Citizens' Initiative – Official Register. "Water and sanitation are a human right! Water is a public good, not a commodity!", registered 10 May 2012.

15 European Commission (2014). *Communication* from the Commission on the European Citizens' Initiative "Water and sanitation are a human right! Water is a public good, not a commodity!" Brussels, released on 19 March 2014.

16 European Commission (2017). The European Citizens' Initiative – Official Register. "Ban glyphosate and protect people and the environment from toxic pesticides", registered 25 January 2017.

17 *Communication* from the Commission on the European Citizens' Initiative, "Ban glyphosate and protect people and the environment from toxic pesticides". Brussels, released on 12 December 2017.

18 European Commission (2018). Proposal for a regulation of the European Parliament and of the Council on the transparency and sustainability of the EU risk assessment in the food chain. Brussels, 11 April 2018.

evaluation of pesticides for EU approval is based only on published studies that are not commissioned by the pesticides industry"). The European Parliament and the Council reached a provisional agreement on the Commission's proposal in February 2019. Although only partially successful, these ECIs have impacted the EU health policy-making process.[19]

The Commission also has a role as the "guardian of the treaties". This means that it is authorized to file cases against Member States that are not in compliance with EU law. The associated procedures involve tracking the transposition of EU legislation into Member State law and warning Member States that the Commission considers it to be failing in the transposition or implementation of EU law. Ultimately the Commission has standing to take Member States to the Court of Justice of the European Union over failure to implement and obey EU law. In January 2019, for instance, the Commission sent letters of formal notice to Austria and the Netherlands, requesting the Austrian and Dutch authorities to comply with the rules on the level of reimbursement laid out in the EU Cross-border Healthcare Directive (Directive 2011/24/EU)[20]. Regarding air quality, the Commission called on France and Sweden to bring their air quality legislation in line with European rules on ambient air quality and cleaner air for Europe (Directive 2008/50/EC).

The legislative processes and the voting procedures that underwrite them (qualified majority voting (QMV) and reverse qualified majority voting (RQMV)) are outlined in Box 2.2.

Finally, the Commission's Structural Reform Support Service (SRSS) helps Member States create and carry out growth-enhancing reforms and as of 2019 is to become a DG in its own right. Established in July 2015, the SRSS coordinates and provides tailor-made support to EU countries in various areas, including healthcare and long-term care systems, governance and public administration, education and climate change. At the request of a national government, the Commission's SRSS discusses technical support needs, agrees to a "cooperation and support plan" with the Member State, provides financing for the support and coordinates experts from the public and private sectors. The SRSS's support is provided through the Structural Reform Support Programme (SRSP), established by Regulation (EU) 2017/825[21] in May 2017 for the period 2017–2020. With

---

19 European Commission (2019). Press release: "Boosting trust in scientific studies on food safety: Commission welcomes the provisional agreement reached today". Brussels, released 11 February 2019.

20 European Commission (2019). Fact Sheet. "January infringements package: key decisions". Brussels, 24 January 2019.

21 Regulation (EU) 2017/825 of the European Parliament and of the Council of 17 May 2017 on the establishment of the Structural Reform Support Programme for the period 2017 to 2020 and amending Regulations (EU) No. 1303/2013 and (EU) No. 1305/2013.

Box 2.2   *EU legislative processes*

The "ordinary legislative procedure", also known as "co-decision", is the general rule for adopting legislation at the EU level. It applies in 85 defined policy areas, which cover most of the EU's areas of competence. This procedure is essentially a similar procedure to most national Parliaments, with a proposal that goes through two readings alternating between two chambers (in this case, the European Parliament and the Council of Ministers), which must reach agreement for the proposal to be adopted.

The Commission holds the right of initiative. The "ordinary legislative procedure" starts therefore with a Commission legislative proposal. The proposal is sent to the Parliament, which may amend it in a "first reading". The Commission's proposal is simultaneously sent to national parliaments, which may issue a "reasoned opinion" stating why they think the draft legislative act does not comply with the principle of subsidiarity (in accordance with Protocol No. 1 on the role of national parliaments and Protocol No. 2 on the principles of subsidiarity and proportionality).

The amended proposal then goes to the Council, which may amend the Parliament's proposal in its own first reading. If they agree, then they can both pass it and it becomes law. If they do not agree, the legislation will pass through a second reading in both, which is quite common. The co-legislators can agree on a compromise text, and then complete the legislative procedure, at any reading. These agreements are reached through inter-institutional negotiations known as "tripartite meetings" or "trilogues" between the EU Parliament, the Council and the Commission.* Trilogues consist mostly of political negotiations, although they may be preceded by technical meetings. Any agreement reached in a trilogue is provisional. It must then be approved through the formal procedures applicable within each institution. The number of trilogues depends on the debated draft proposal and specific political circumstances. The institutionalized use of trilogues seems to have strengthened transparency and accountability within the Parliament.**

Trilogues have also changed the actual operation of the political process; by coordinating the institutions early in the process, they smooth the path to legislation but reduce the number of initiatives proposed that do not pass. Whether trilogues will continue to work that way as the political factions in the Council and Parliament continue to fragment remains to be seen.

If the Council second reading does not approve the amendments from the Parliament's second reading, a "conciliation committee" of MEPs and Council representatives tries to formulate a compromise. If they formulate a proposal and both the Parliament and the Council pass it unamended, then it becomes law; if they fail to agree on a proposal or it is not passed by Council or Parliament, then the legislative proposal has failed. This process is used for most legislation relevant to health.

The Parliament has a majority voting rule: a majority of MEPs wins a vote. The Council has more complex voting rules that depend on the issue. Simple majority is a simple majority of Member

States (15 being a majority at the moment). The qualified majority voting rules (QMV) require votes from at least 16 Member States. The proposal must be supported by Member States representing at least 65% of the total EU population. Some issues, such as regulation of social security (which includes the European Health Insurance Card) require unanimity in the Council. Fiscal governance issues sometimes require the newest voting rule, reverse qualified majority voting, in which a qualified majority is required to reject the Commission proposal; this is a rule designed to strengthen the Commission. The treaties spell out the voting rules for each issue. The treaties include a *passerelle* clause allowing voting rules to be changed from special to the ordinary legislative procedure, or to replace unanimity rules with QMV.

How to follow negotiations between the EU institutions

The European Parliament provides a "Legislative Observatory" (http://www.europarl.europa.eu/oeil/home/home.do) to enable the process of a particular legislative proposal to be followed in detail. The process can be followed in all the institutions from the Commission's initial proposal, and the current position can be seen. With some knowledge of the decision-making processes of the institutions, this provides an excellent overview and access to the individual documents and positions along the way.

* European Parliament. "Handbook on the Ordinary Legislative Procedure. A guide to how the European Parliament co-legislates". Available at: http://www.epgencms.europarl.europa.eu/cmsdata/upload/10fc26a9-7f3e-4d8a-a46d-51bdadc9661c/handbook-olp-en.pdf, accessed 4 June 2019.

** *Idem* p. 29.

an initial budget of €142.8 million[22] (2017–2020) and an additional budget of €80 million approved in September 2018 for the period 2019–2020, the SRSP provides extensive support to all Member States. Examples of support provided in the healthcare arena include primary healthcare reforms (Austria), cancer screening programmes (Italy, Slovakia and Romania), health system performance assessment (Latvia and Slovenia), spending review on medicines, functional integration of hospitals, etc.[23] In Italy, Romania and Slovakia the national health authorities submitted a request for support to the Commission in 2017. The SRSS helped them improve the implementation of EU colorectal cancer screening guidelines, through the training and empowering of senior health managers and health professionals, developing communication campaigns, organizing country visits, etc. Austria also requested support from SRSS, in order to speed up the implementation of a primary healthcare reform the country had previously adopted to establish 75 primary healthcare units by 2022. The SRSS created a website, a communication strategy and support material to enable health

22 European Commission. "European Commission Structural Reform Support Service" website: https://ec.europa.eu/info/sites/info/files/srss-information-brochure_en.pdf.

23 European Commission (2018). Structural Support Reform Service. "Current Activities and Plan for a future Reform Support Service". Luxembourg, 28 September 2018. Available at: https://ec.europa.eu/health/sites/health/files/non_communicable_diseases/docs/ev_20180928_co07_en.pdf.

professionals to start their own primary healthcare unit. The Commission's SRSS is therefore a new but effective power player.

2.1.2 European Parliament

The first EU legislative chamber is the European Parliament, which has been gaining power since its establishment in the 1970s. Although initially very much the junior partner within the legislature, the Parliament now acts as co-legislator with the Council of Ministers in nearly all areas. The Parliament is elected by direct vote across Europe for a five-year term and organized into party groups that largely resemble the party groupings of most Member States. No single political group has a majority within the Parliament, and so decision-making in practice requires considerable collaboration across political groups.

Box 2.3   *Political groups in the 2019–2024 European Parliament and percentage of members*

Group of the European People's Party (Christian Democrats): 24.23%

Group of the Progressive Alliance of Socialists and Democrats: 20.51%

Renew Europe: 14.38%

Groups of the Greens/European Free Alliance: 9.85%

Europe of Nations and Freedom Group now known as Identity and Democracy: 9.72%

European Conservatives and Reformists Group: 8.26%

Confederal Group of the European United Left/Nordic Green Left: 5.46%

Non-Attached Members 7.59%

Over time, the Parliament has been gaining power, with more and more areas subject to ordinary legislative procedure (also known as co-decisions; *see* Box 2.2), with increased powers over the budget, the power to hold hearings on a variety of issues and question commissioners, and the ability to veto candidates for Commission President as put forth by the Council.

In practical terms, the Parliament works principally through 20 standing committees for the different policy areas, with the committee responsible for the subject of a proposal taking the lead in the Parliament's consideration of it. The lead committee for health issues is the Environment, Public Health and Food Safety Committee (ENVI), although other committees also play a significant role in relation to health, such as the Employment and Social Affairs Committee (which deals with social security coordination, for example), or the Industry, Research and Energy Committee (which deals with research on health). In terms of process for a given proposal, an individual MEP within the committee concerned is nominated to prepare a report on behalf of the Parliament; this member is termed the *rapporteur* for the proposal. This report is then considered and revised by the committee as a whole, and then by Parliament as a whole in one of the monthly plenary sessions.

For the first time since direct elections to the European Parliament began in 1979, the two largest groups – the Group of the European People's Party (EPP) and the Group of the Progressive Alliance of Socialists and Democrats (S&D) – have lost their combined majority in the Parliament in the 2019 European elections. Their partnership, known as the "Grand coalition", held 54% of the seats before the vote but is now down to 45% of the seats. S&D won 154 seats (20.51%) while EPP won 182 seats (24.23%), out of 751 seats.[24] Other parties made substantial gains, including the Group of the Alliance of Liberals and Democrats for Europe + Renaissance + USR (ALDE&R), now Renew Europe, with 108 seats (14.38%), the Group of the Greens/European Free Alliance (ECR) with 74 seats (9.85%), up from 52 seats in 2014. Right wing nationalist and Eurosceptic groups also saw gains. This more fragmented European Parliament, which mirrors the more fragmented political systems of most Member States, creates new political and coalitional possibilities, might change the way trilogues operate (Box 2.2), and makes the EU agenda less predictable.

2.1.3 Council of Ministers and the European Council

The second EU legislative body is the Council of Ministers. This is made up of the relevant ministers from each Member State meeting in one of ten topic-specific configurations (e.g. a Health Council will be composed of the ministers responsible for health);[25] indeed, a Member State may be represented by several different ministers during the course of a single Council meeting, depending on the subjects being discussed. This structure is unlike any national government, where there is a single body for multiple policies: although technically one body, in practice the Council for Agriculture and Fisheries is not made up of the same national representatives as the Council for Employment, Social Policy, Health and Consumer Affairs. This approach relies on effective coordination at national level to ensure that the positions expressed in one Council take account of the full

---

24 https://www.election-results.eu.

25 *See* Council of the European Union (2019). *Council configurations*. Brussels, Council of the European Union. Available at: https://www.consilium.europa.eu/en/council-eu/configurations/, accessed 2 May 2019.

Table 2.1 *Order of presidencies of the Council of Ministers*

Period	Country	Period	Country
2019 (first half)	Romania	2025 (first half)	Poland
2019 (second half)	Finland	2025 (second half)	Denmark
2020 (first half)	Croatia	2026 (first half)	Cyprus
2020 (second half)	Germany	2026 (second half)	Ireland
2021 (first half)	Portugal	2027 (first half)	Lithuania
2021 (second half)	Slovenia	2027 (second half)	Greece
2022 (first half)	France	2028 (first half)	Italy
2022 (second half)	Czech Republic	2028 (second half)	Latvia
2023 (first half)	Sweden	2029 (first half)	Luxembourg
2023 (second half)	Spain	2029 (second half)	Netherlands
2024 (first half)	Belgium	2030 (first half)	Slovakia
2024 (second half)	Hungary	2030 (second half)	Malta

range of views domestically (e.g. if health-related expenditure is being discussed in the Economic and Financial Affairs Council). Given that the Member States (and indeed the Commission) face the usual coordination problems of big bureaucracies and handle them with variable success,[26] the result is that a level of fragmentation exists in the heart of the EU legislative process.

In the Council, coordination is in the hands of the Council Presidency. A pivotal role is that of chairing Council meetings, setting their agenda and brokering compromises. The responsibility for doing this is shared among all the EU countries, with each country taking a six-month stint to hold the Presidency of the Council (Table 2.1).[27] The Council has an intricate but broadly majority-type voting system, although in practice the Council aims to seek consensus wherever possible. Most European legislation, including health legislation, requires the agreement of both the Parliament and the Council. Both the Council and the Parliament can also agree political statements, which are not legally enforceable but which clearly state priorities and policies. The Council can also adopt *Recommendations*; these are legal acts but without any legal mechanism of enforcement. Nevertheless, the political weight of such a commitment is substantial, and they have proved effective in the health area on subjects such as cancer screening.[28]

---

26 The classic articulation of the problem is seen in Wright V (1996). "The national co-ordination of European policy-making: negotiating the quagmire", in Richardson JJ (ed.). *European Union: power and policy-making*. London: Routledge; also Greer SL (2010). Standing up for health? Health departments in the making of EU policy. *Social Policy and Administration*, 44(2):208–24.

27 Council of the European Union (2007). Decision of 1 January 2007 determining the order in which the office of President of the Council shall be held. *Official Journal*, L 1/11.

28 Council of the European Union (2003). Recommendation of 2 December 2003 on cancer screening. *Official Journal*, L 327/34.

The European Council is made up of the heads of state and government of the Member States; this is formally a separate body from the Council of Ministers (and cannot adopt legislation, for example), but as it is made up of the most powerful political figures in Europe, it has a leadership role in setting the overall direction of the EU and brokering solutions to its most intractable problems. Unlike the rotating Presidency of the Council of Ministers, the European Council has an elected president. The first elected President of the Council was Belgian Christian Democrat and former prime minister Herman van Rompuy. Donald Tusk, former Prime Minister of Poland from the European People's Party member Civil Coalition, replaced him on 1 December 2014. Belgian liberal and former prime minister Charles Michel will replace Tusk in 2019.

There is a variety of types of EU legal instrument specified in the treaties, and the differences between them are legally and politically significant (Box 2.4).

2.1.4 Court of Justice of the European Union

Finally, the EU has a court, the CJEU. Formerly known as the European Court of Justice, it is the most powerful supranational court in history.[29] It is made up of judges nominated by the Member States, sitting in Luxembourg. It is the final arbiter of EU law; if Member States disagree with the CJEU on legal interpretation, they must change the law, and if they disagree with its interpretation of treaties, they must change the treaties.

EU law is an impressive edifice, built by both the CJEU and the courts of the Member States interpreting EU law in the course of deciding cases on the correct interpretation of EU law (Box 2.5). EU law has both direct effect, meaning that it is directly applicable in Member States even if the Member State has not transposed it into domestic legislation, and supremacy, meaning that it overrides Member State law (with only a few qualifications, every EU Member State court has accepted both of these doctrines). EU institutions can bring cases directly to the CJEU, as when the Commission sues Member States for failure to correctly implement legislation, but many CJEU cases come about because of litigation in a Member State that raises a question of EU law. The Member States' courts may interpret EU law as well as their domestic laws, and they may use the "preliminary reference procedure" to refer the question to the CJEU for clarification (article 267 of the TFEU). The CJEU ruling is then case law, binding until overridden by legislation, a treaty change or new CJEU case law. Much of the history of healthcare law in the EU has involved the CJEU making rulings under the preliminary reference procedure when courts in Member States have faced cases brought by people who wished to use healthcare outside their home

---

29 Stone Sweet A (2005). "Judicial authority and market integration in Europe", in Ginsburg T & Kagan RA (eds.). *Institutions and public law: comparative approaches*. Frankfurt: Peter Lang.

Box 2.4   *Commonly used terms in EU law*

Regulations and directives

Regulations and directives are the EU's principal legal instruments. A regulation, once passed, is directly applicable: it becomes Member State law, in the words passed at the EU level. In health, a key regulation of relevance is that on the coordination of social security systems, which also includes provisions on people receiving healthcare in other Member States (section 4.3.1). Regulations are also used to establish agencies, such as the European Medicines Agency. A directive is EU legislation that Member States must transpose into their own domestic law. It sets out the objectives to be achieved but leaves it up to Member States as to how they achieve those objectives in their national context.

Decisions

A decision is binding on its addresses within specific legislative areas and can do a variety of things, such as ratify Commission reports (as in the European Semester).

Recommendations and declarative documents

Recommendations are legal acts but have no binding force. The institutions also adopt various types of declarative document (principally *Communications* from the Commission, *Conclusions* from the Council and *Opinions* from the Parliament); these also have no binding force but shape the agenda. Council *Recommendations* and *Resolutions* have more force than Conclusions. The Commission, in particular, strongly prefers to have authorization from such a document for its proposals and activities, even if Member States and outsiders might complain that what the Commission is doing is not what they intended.[a]

Delegation

Detailed primary legislation is not always appropriate (e.g. in areas where there are frequent technical changes) and so EU legislation adopted by the Council and Parliament frequently delegates powers to the Commission to adopt subsidiary measures under the main legislation. This is subject to scrutiny by the Member States (typically through the Commission consulting a committee of Member State representatives before adopting a subsidiary measure) and the European Parliament. Before the Lisbon Treaty, the system of delegated powers for the Commission and the controls over them was generally set out in the "comitology" decision of the Council.[b] This provided for a range of different procedures with differing degrees of oversight from the Council (and the Parliament, though less so). The Lisbon Treaty aimed to simplify these procedures, reducing what had become quite a wide range of ways in which powers could be delegated.

It replaced the previous systems of delegated powers with two types of delegated power. These are described in the treaty itself:[c]

Delegated acts: where the Commission is given *"the power to adopt non-legislative acts of general application to supplement or amend certain non-essential elements of the legislative act. The objectives, content, scope and duration of the delegation of power shall be explicitly defined in the legislative acts. The essential elements of an area shall be reserved for the legislative act and accordingly shall not be the subject of a delegation of power."* – Article 290 of the Treaty on the Functioning of the European Union. Unlike previous procedures, no formal committee of Member State representatives is required, although the Commission is committed to consulting "experts from the national authorities of all the Member States, which will be responsible for implementing the delegated acts once they have been adopted";[d]

Implementing acts: *"Where uniform conditions for implementing legally binding Union acts are needed, those acts shall confer implementing powers on the Commission, or, in duly justified specific cases and in the cases provided for in Articles 24 and 26 of the Treaty on European Union, on the Council."* – Article 291 TFEU. Two specific procedures for how the Commission consults a committee of Member States' representatives for implementing acts have been set out in Regulation (EU) 182/2011,[e] a lighter "advisory" procedure and a stricter "examination" procedure; any implementing act affecting the health or safety of humans must follow the stricter "examination" procedure.[f]

In practice, what this means is that in addition to the formal and high-profile processes of law-making that take place through the Council and the Parliament, there is also a much less visible process of adopting secondary acts. Even though these are only secondary legislation, they can involve decisions that can be highly significant for those affected by the relevant primary legislation.

An alternative legislative method allows the *social partners*, sectoral representatives of employers and labour, to negotiate legislation with each other and have it become law for their sector. In health, this has produced one piece of legislation: a Directive on sharps (e.g. safe handling of needles and other products that can pose a hazard to workers).[g]

---

[a] Page EC (2012). "The European Commission bureaucracy: handling sovereignty through the back and front doors", in Hayward J & Wurzel R (eds.). *European disunion: between sovereignty and solidarity*. Basingstoke: Palgrave Macmillan.

[b] *See* Council Decision 1999/468/EC, *Official Journal*, L 184 of 17 July 1999.

[c] For a more detailed guide *see* Hardacre A, Kaeding (2013). *Delegated & implementing acts: The new comitology.* 5th ed. Maastricht, the Netherlands: European Institute of Public Administration (EIPA).

[d] *See* COM(2009)673.

[e] *Official Journal*, L 55 of 28 February 2011.

[f] *See* Article 2(b)(iii).

[g] Council of the European Union. Directive 2010/32/EU: prevention from sharp injuries in the hospital and healthcare sector of 10 May 2010 implementing the Framework Agreement on prevention from sharp injuries in the hospital and healthcare sector concluded by HOSPEEM and EPSU. Brussels: Council of the European Union.

country.[30] As with most courses, the CJEU has also learned about the sector through the cases it sees, and it is possible to read its jurisprudence as a process of learning how to adapt internal market principles to the specific politics and issues in healthcare.[31]

The accession to the European Union of new states with different healthcare systems raises uncertainties regarding the applicability of EU health laws.[32] National courts have used the preliminary reference procedure to seek answers through the CJEU. In *Georgi Ivanov Elchinov v. Natsionalna zdravnoosiguritelna kasa*, for instance, a Bulgarian Administrative Court asked the CJEU whether a "national court (is) obliged to take account of binding directions given to it by a higher court when its decision is set aside and the case referred back for reconsideration if there is reason to assume that such directions are inconsistent with Community law".[33] The Bulgarian court also asked the CJEU about the payment of costs incurred in a hospital located in another EU Member State (Germany), because the patient could not materially receive treatment in his home country, Bulgaria, where there is an alternative treatment, which is both less effective and more radical than the treatment available in Germany.[34]

Regarding the first issue, the CJEU ruled that "lower courts whose decisions were set aside by a higher court could, relying on that case-law, and when the case was referred back to them, disregard the setting-aside of their judgment by the higher court when, in their opinion, it was contrary to European Union law. In the conflict between national procedural autonomy and the opportunity, which was thus reopened, to assert the primacy of European Union law, priority was given to the latter" (Point 21). Regarding the second issue, the CJEU ruled that prior authorization may be refused if the medical benefits provided abroad are not covered under the patient's social security system. However, if the treatment method applied abroad corresponds to benefits covered in the patient's Member State, it is not permissible to refuse prior authorization on the ground that such a method is not practised in that Member State.[35]

30 Obermaier AJ (2008). The national judiciary: sword of European Court of Justice rulings – the example of the Kohll/Decker jurisprudence. *European Law Journal*, 14(6):735–52.

31 Martinsen DS (2015). *An ever more powerful court?: The political constraints of legal integration in the European Union*. Oxford: Oxford University Press.

32 Stanislas A, Cheynel B, Rolin F (2015). La Cour de justice, acteur multifonctionnel du développement du droit économique de l'Union, *Revue internationale de droit économique*, 2015:4.

33 CJEU (2010). Judgment of the Court (Grand Chamber) of 5 October 2010, *Georgi Ivanov Elchinov v Natsionalna zdravnoosiguritelna kasa*.

34 Court of Justice of the European Union. "The Court of Justice and healthcare" website. Available at: https://curia.europa.eu/jcms/upload/docs/application/pdf/2018-11/qd-04-18-747-en-n.pdf, accessed 10 June 2019.

35 Greer SL, Sokol T (2014). Rules for Rights: European Law, Health Care and Social Citizenship. *European Law Journal*, 20(1):66–87; Sokol T (2010). *Rindal* and *Elchinov*: A (n) (Impending) Revolution in EU Law on Patient Mobility? *Croatian Yearbook of European Law and Policy*, 6(6):167–208.

Box 2.5 *Key concepts in European integration*

Creating an integrated Europe through implementing free movement of goods, services, capital and people is an awesome legal and policy-making task. The EU has developed a series of legal principles and techniques that it uses to carry on its task. Viewed together, they are a toolkit for creating both a powerful legal system and an increasingly integrated market and society. There are several key legal tools and concepts.

Harmonization. This refers to setting EU standards for something in place of diverging national standards (e.g. basic requirements for the number of hours that constitute medical education).

Mutual recognition. EU Member States, even if their regulations differ, agree to recognize the quality of the regulations in other EU Member States and not discriminate against goods, services, capital or people regulated by another Member State. It is often used with a measure of harmonization that sets the floor.[a] For example, the EU has mutual recognition of medical qualifications combined with limited harmonization of the requirements for achieving those qualifications. The virtue of mutual recognition is that it spares the EU from having to legislate detailed standards for everything in the EU (e.g. the full set of requirements to be a doctor in Europe), which would be time-consuming if not impossible. The potential drawback is that it depends on very different Member States having equally good regulation, and gives Member States very few responses if the floor is set too low in EU law or another Member State has less stringent standards or enforcement. Since most legislation is adopted under QMV, Member States will have had chances to influence it but might not have been in agreement with it.

Country of origin principle. This is similar to the mutual recognition scheme. It states that a service or product acceptable in one country must be accepted in another. While the country of origin principle has no explicit legal basis in the treaties, it forms part of the foundations of the internal market. The country of origin principle was exemplified in a legal dispute between France and Germany on the alcoholic beverage *Cassis de Dijon.*[b]

Direct effect. Individuals may rely on rights provided by EU law directly (under certain circumstances), whether or not their Member State has taken measures to incorporate that EU law into their domestic legislation. A legal doctrine developed by the CJEU, it means that even if a state fails to transpose a directive into law or enforce it, citizens can use the EU law as a basis for litigation, provided that certain conditions are met (in particular that the rights concerned are clear, unconditional and do not require additional measures).

Precedence. The CJEU has also developed the doctrine of precedence, meaning that EU law is superior to Member States' law, and if a Member State law contradicts EU law, then the EU law is what shall be applied.

Subsidiarity. Balancing all of this integrative apparatus is the concept of subsidiarity, which is that tasks should be performed at the smallest unit possible. Usually, this is taken to mean that the EU should not do things that the Member States could do better; whether Member

States choose to go on and decentralize themselves is their business.

Decentralized enforcement of EU law.   Finally, the EU relies principally on the Member States for decentralized enforcement of its law. Direct effect and precedence mean that individual citizens or companies can bring challenges. So, even if the Commission does not start a court case against a Member State for some form of non-compliance, those affected by the law can often bring cases themselves. If their Member State courts see an issue of lack of clarity in applicable EU law, they can use the preliminary reference procedure to ask the CJEU's opinion. This is how a single case of a citizen or a company with a problem can go via Member State courts to the CJEU and influence or use EU law even if no elected official supports the citizen or company's case. It needs to be acknowledged that rulings by the CJEU, even though they are directed towards individual cases, establish principles and case law that has to be respected throughout the EU in the interpretation and application of EU law.

---

^a   Nicolaidis K (2005). "Globalization with a human face: managed mutual recognition and the free movement of professionals", in Kostoris F & Schioppa P (eds.). *The principle of mutual recognition in the European integration process.* Basingstoke: Palgrave Macmillan.

^b   European Court of Justice. Case C-120/78 *Cassis de Dijon.*

2.1.5   Other treaty bodies: European Central Bank, European Investment Bank, Economic and Social Committee, Committee of the Regions, European Court of Auditors, and the Ombudsman

The European Central Bank (ECB), although not part of the EU legislative process, is particularly important as it is the central bank of the Eurozone. It has a high level of autonomy entrenched in treaties that also give it specific obligations, notably to keep inflation low, and constraints, including a prohibition on making loans to EU institutions or Member States. Its leadership is made up of an Executive Board, whose six members are appointed by the Council under QMV; a Governing Council, made up of the Executive Board and the Member States' central bank heads of the Eurozone; and a General Council, made up of the Executive Board and the heads of all the EU central banks. All have security of tenure and may not be reappointed; by law, they must be politically independent.

On paper, the ECB has a narrowly limited remit that has little to do with health. In practice, it is very powerful and can shape health policy. The logic of increasing the predictability of central banks by decreasing their accountability to others has the obvious flaw that the unaccountable can be unpredictable.[36] The ECB demonstrated this over the decade since the financial crisis began, with unconventional monetary policy whose relationship to its mission could

---

36   Adolph C (2013). *Bankers, bureaucrats and central bank politics: the myth of neutrality.* Cambridge: Cambridge University Press.

be unclear, and its participation in the "Troika" using conditional lending to reform Cyprus, Greece, Ireland and Portugal, and to a lesser extent Spain and Italy, was quite novel in the history of central banking.[37] Likewise, interventions by the ECB and its member banks in the domestic politics of Italy and Greece were not clearly justified in the treaties. Regardless of the legitimacy and effect of these interventions, they were certainly consequential for health.

In July 2019 Christine Lagarde, former finance minister of France and managing director of the IMF, was appointed president of the ECB.

The European Investment Bank (EIB) (*see* section 5.3.4) provides funding for projects that seek to achieve EU goals, within or outside the European Union. It has, over the last decade, increased its exposure to health and sought to improve the sophistication of its lending, in particular to health systems.

In addition to the ECB and the EIB, the European Court of Auditors (ECA) was established in 1977 to audit the EU's finances. As the EU's independent external auditor, the ECA is responsible for checking if the EU budget has been implemented correctly and if EU funds have been spent legally and in accordance with EU public finance regulations. The Court of Auditors has been making an increasing number of interventions into the health arena, focusing on misjudged policies and mis-spent money. Most recently, it evaluated the impact of the directive on cross-border patient mobility (*see* section 4.3.1).[38] In general, its reports are well done, even if they can be very awkward for the rest of the institutions.

In the same vein, the European Ombudsman is a person elected by the European Parliament under Article 228 with a mission to "receive complaints from any citizen of the Union or any natural or legal person residing or having its registered office in a Member State concerning instances of maladministration in the activities of the Union institutions, bodies, offices or agencies, with the exception of the Court of Justice of the European Union acting in its judicial role. He or she shall examine such complaints and report on them." The Ombudsman's term coincides with that of the European Parliament. The outgoing Ombudsman (2014–2019), Emily O'Reilly, has proved adept at using the position to raise inconvenient questions about decision-making processes.[39] At the end of 2019,

---

37 Greer SL, Jarman H (2016). "Reinforcing Europe's failed fiscal regulatory state" in Dallago B, Guri G & McGowan J (eds.). *A Global Perspective on the European Economic Crisis*. London: Routledge, pp. 122–43; Fahy N (2012). Who is shaping the future of European health systems? *BMJ*, 13;344:e1712.

38 Special report no. 07/2019: EU actions for cross-border healthcare: significant ambitions but improved management required. European Court of Auditors. July 2019. Available at: https://www.eca.europa.eu/en/Pages/DocItem.aspx?did=49945.

39 Lee M (2015). "Accountability and Co-Production Beyond Courts: The Role of the European Ombudsman", in Weimer M & de Ruijter A (eds.). *Regulating Risks in the European Union: The co-production of Expert and Executive Power*. Hart Publishing, pp. 217–40.

for example, the Ombudsman opened an inquiry into corporate sponsorship of EU Council presidencies, including the Finnish presidency's links with car maker BMW and the Romanian presidency's sponsorship by Coca-Cola.[40] It was responding to a complaint by a civil society organization, Foodwatch International, which singled out the contribution of Coca-Cola's products to obesity and diabetes.[41]

Finally, the EU legislative process also includes the Economic and Social Committee, which represents social partners (employers and workers), and the Committee of the Regions, which agglomerates the opinions of subnational governments (and which the Commission sometimes uses to get a sense of how regional governments feel about legislative proposals). Both are strictly advisory, although consultation with them is mandatory in some areas of policy specified in the treaties.

2.1.6   Agencies

Beyond the central institutions of the EU, there is also a constellation of specialist EU agencies created to carry out specific tasks. There are many of relevance to health policy, including the European Centre for Disease Prevention and Control (ECDC), the European Food Safety Authority (EFSA), the European Medicines Agency (EMA), the European Monitoring Centre for Drugs and Drug Addiction (EMCDDA),[42] the European Environment Agency (EEA) and the European Agency for Safety & Health at Work (OSHA). With a slightly different legal status, there is also the Consumers, Health, Agriculture and Food Executive Agency (CHAFEA), formerly the European Agency for Health and Consumers, to which the Commission has delegated the implementation of health programmes.[43]

These agencies are part of a large set of EU agencies working in technical areas. Their common denominator is that they are established by EU regulations, and their power is limited to the specific activities delegated to them in the legal act establishing them. At their most powerful, as with EFSA and EMA, they make

---

40   Letter to the Secretary-General of the Council of the European Union, Mr Jeppe Tranholm-Mikkelsen, concerning commercial sponsorship of Presidencies. 14 July 2019. Case 1069/2019/MIG.

41   Foodwatch International (2019). Foodwatch demands end of EU-presidency partnership with Coca-Cola. Available at: https://www.foodwatch.org/en/news/2019/foodwatch-demands-end-of-eu-presidency-partnership-with-coca-cola/.

42   Urrestarazu A et al. (2019). Brexit threatens the UK's ability to tackle illicit drugs and organised crime: What needs to happen now? *Health Policy*, 123(6):521–5.

43   European Commission. CHAFEA, EU Health Programme website. Available at: http://ec.europa.eu/chafea/health/index_en.htm, accessed 1 May 2019. CHAFEA administers a range of EU grants and contracts in the general area of health and social policy. Unlike the other agencies listed, it lacks its own legal status and is essentially an administrative function of the Commission.

technical assessments of issues such as medicine safety or food nutritional claims, and then control the documentation and access to market of different products.

The case for agencies in the EU is in large part the same as the case for agencies elsewhere. Agencies are partially freed from the staffing limits and changing priorities of the central civil service (in this case, the Commission) and can hire and retain technical experts. Their focus and physical distance from Brussels make them more technocratic and, if not less political, at least less embroiled in the day-to-day politics of the EU. The governing regulations of the agencies give them clear and circumscribed missions, which means that they can be trusted to carry out their tasks with a limit on their political engagement. Rightly or wrongly, Member States often express the view that the Commission will use any resources or mandates to expand its power.[44] Agencies' governing boards form an extra level of control for Member States, and the composition of the boards matters and varies a great deal. Agencies with large boards (e.g. with representatives from every Member State) might have informed stakeholders but such unwieldy boards will often allow great autonomy to executives. As a result of their attributes – predictability, technical focus and autonomy within limits – agencies have been a popular tool of EU action (although more so with national governments than with the European Parliament, which has raised doubts about its lack of oversight of agencies) and are particularly densely concentrated in technical areas such as the safety of chemicals or aviation, where details are complex, intricate, not particularly visible in daily life and prone to cause crises when they are not handled well.

In political terms, a key limitation of these agencies is that they have no ability to propose changes to any of the legislation that they help to oversee; any such proposals still have to be made by the Commission. This means that such agencies may well be seen as technically authoritative, but they are not direct actors in the EU decision-making processes.

Another part of the appeal of EU agencies to national governments has been that they are distributed around the Union, rather than being based in Brussels. As well as distributing the benefits of jobs and economic activity more widely, countries have argued that they can provide particularly appropriate homes for certain agencies, such as through synergies with particular domestic facilities. How much difference the specific geographical location of an EU agency really makes to either the agency or its host country has been unclear but is about to get some empirical tests, with the move of the European Medicines Agency from London to Amsterdam, and the move of the European Banking Authority to Paris. How far related activity also follows these moves will be an interesting

---

44 Pollack MA (2003). *The engines of European integration: delegation, agency, and agenda setting in the EU.* Oxford: Oxford University Press.

gauge of how valuable it is to have an EU agency in your country, and will doubtless be closely watched.

2.1.7   How do EU institutions take account of the EU's indirect impact on health?

The question this leaves is: how do the key actors in the EU make sure that as European action is developed and implemented, the EU understands the effect it is having on health and guides its action accordingly?

The Commission's answer has been discussed above. There is a high degree of internal coordination before policies are proposed (although whether this is always fully effective is a matter of debate; and as it is part of internal processes which are not public, the trade-offs made are not transparent to the outside).[45]

The Parliament has explicit mechanisms for incorporating different perspectives within its process; if several different committees all have an interest in a file, they have an opportunity to be consulted and put forward amendments for their areas of responsibility. Where disagreements remain, these can be taken to the full plenary session of Parliament and sorted out there.[46] Moreover, as the various meetings, amendments and discussions of the Parliament are public, it is much easier to understand what interests have been taken into account and how they have been balanced.

The Council, however, takes a different approach and one that gives rise to particular tensions. Although the Council meets in different thematic formations (see section 2.1.3), it does not allow a Council with one thematic focus (such as health) to comment or otherwise engage with the decisions being taken by another (such as economic affairs). This means that a wide range of decisions will be decided upon in the Council by ministers other than health ministers. The logic behind this is that Member State governments should do their coordination at home and whoever represents the government in Brussels should be able to present an integrated opinion. However, this is not always equally effective, and for a subject such as health it can be very frustrating for national health ministers to find that they have no way to express themselves directly in Brussels on most of the decisions that affect them (*see* chapter 5). In an attempt to increase transparency and policy coherence, the concept of a "roadmap" has been established (Box 2.4).[47]

---

45 Ståhl T et al. (eds.) (2006). *Health in all policies: prospects and potentials*. Helsinki: Ministry of Social Affairs and Health.

46 European Parliament. *Rules of procedure of the European Parliament*. Brussels: European Parliament. Available at: http://www.europarl.europa.eu/sides/getLastRules.do?language=EN&reference=TOC, accessed 4 July 2014.

47 Roadmaps are available at https://ec.europa.eu/smart-regulation/roadmaps/index_en.htm.

2.2 Budget

The constitutional asymmetry of the EU is particularly visible in its limited finances. Overall government expenditure tends to be around 50% of gross domestic product (GDP) across the EU, but this is overwhelmingly spent within the Member States themselves; in 2018 the EU itself had a budget capped at around 0.84% of the EU's gross national product (Fig. 2.1). Within the budget, the biggest area of expenditure is the agricultural budget (€59.2 billion in 2018), followed by structural and cohesion funds (€55.5 billion) intended to reduce inequalities in development across the EU, and the EU's research programme (€11.2 billion) (Fig. 2.2). These three areas account for over 82% of the EU budget, with other areas (including specific expenditure on healthcare actions) being minor in comparison; EU administration represents €9.6 million.[48] In terms of the major areas of public finances in Europe as a whole, therefore, only in agriculture is European funding predominant; in all other sectors, national (or regional) funding is the principal source, and this is certainly true for health.

Fig. 2.1   *EU budget for 2018 in relation to its GDP*

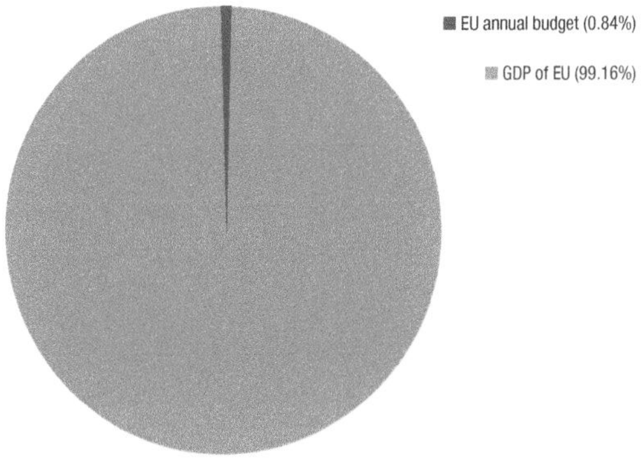

■ EU annual budget (0.84%)

■ GDP of EU (99.16%)

Sources: http://ec.europa.eu/budget/library/biblio/publications/2017/EUbudget-factsheet-2018_en.pdf

In order to avoid annual rows over funding, the EU prefers to have one big argument every seven years and agree an overall allocation of funding for that whole seven-year period. This is called the Multi-annual Financial Framework (MFF). Finland's presidency of the Council of the European Union informed ministers about its plans regarding work on the MFF for 2021–2027 on 18 July 2019. In its June 2019 conclusions, the European Council called on the presidency to develop the MFF's Negotiating Box. On that basis, EU leaders will hold an exchange of views in October, aiming for an agreement before the end of 2019.

---

48   European Commission (2017). 2018 EU Budget. Available at: http://ec.europa.eu/budget/library/biblio/publications/2017/EUbudget-factsheet-2018_en.pdf.

Fig. 2.2   *EU budget for 2018*

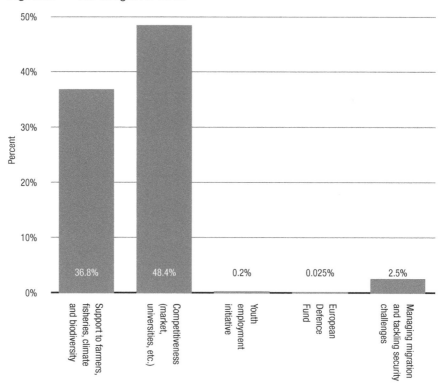

Source: http://ec.europa.eu/budget/library/biblio/publications/2017/EUbudget-factsheet-2018_en.pdf

Although the detailed EU budget is still negotiated and agreed annually, this takes place within the overall Multiannual Financial Framework, and thus these total amounts are unlikely to shift substantially over this period.

There are two important areas of funding specifically allocated to health (structural funds, discussed in section 5.4, often finance health-related projects but are not specifically designed to finance health work). The first, and the one with the highest profile in health policy circles, has historically been the EU health programme. The second is the allocation for health within the research programme of the EU (section 3.7). This is both much larger and more targeted (being only for research), although it is still small in comparison with national expenditure on research, and of course with private expenditure, in particular by the pharmaceutical industry.

2.3   Strengthening legitimacy of EU health policy: civil society and stakeholders

The European Union, in important ways, is unlike any of its Member States. It grew from different roots, born of the complex accommodations needed if such different societies are to work together. It is larger, more fragmented, more complex and does different things in different ways. One result is that the interest group landscapes of the different Member States do not resemble the interest group landscape of the EU. There are different rules, stakeholders and jargon, as well as different problems. Perhaps alarmingly, if the EU lobbying landscape resembles that of any other polity, it is the US that it most resembles.[49] This section discusses some of the interest representation and stakeholders. But it also is a polity that, in lieu of the legitimacy its Member States enjoy, has been particularly attentive to and engaged in developing legitimacy for itself and its policies – becoming, at times, more open and transparent than many states.

2.3.1   Making EU policy legitimate

There are three basic kinds of legitimacy in democratic politics.[50] The EU's search for legitimacy in a crowded political landscape shapes both its choices and its constraints, and makes the institutional analysis of the EU as well as its policy outcomes more intelligible. It also explains the creativity of the EU in developing ways to engage with stakeholders and promote diversity of voices in policy.

Input legitimacy is the legitimacy that comes from democracy: a government is legitimate if created by the people. Most EU Member State governments and their decisions are regarded as legitimate because they were elected in free and fair elections. The EU has had a difficult time gaining input legitimacy for a variety of reasons, ranging from the diversity of its many peoples to its perceived institutional distance from many voters. Direct elections to the European Parliament, the citizens initiative, and the *spitzenkandidat* procedure that elected Jean-Claude Juncker but was abandoned in 2019 are all efforts to give the EU input legitimacy for its actions.

Output legitimacy is the legitimacy that comes from being seen to take creditworthy actions. It is the historical basis for EU legitimacy: that it works. It is what we see in pro-EU arguments that point to Europe-wide mobile phone roaming or low-cost aviation as achievements of the EU. Appeal to output legitimacy has not always worked: some EU actions (e.g. food safety or much environmental law) are so technical that voters do not see them, connect them with outcomes

---

49   Woll C (2008). *Firm interests: How governments shape business lobbying on global trade*. Ithaca, NY: Cornell University Press.

50   Schmidt VA (2013). Democracy and legitimacy in the European Union revisited: Input, output and 'throughput'. *Political Studies*, 61(1):2–22.

or attribute responsibility correctly. Others are unpopular in the short term but beneficial in the longer term, such as many rules about health and safety in the workplace. Member State governments generally try to take credit for popular policies and blame others, including the EU, for less attractive results. Even the most directly visible kind of EU action, structural funds with their obligatory EU symbols, do not always produce the magnitude of legitimacy that one might expect (as we see from popular anti-EU sentiment in areas that have received considerable EU funds, notably in the UK and Central and Eastern Europe (CEE) states). Output legitimacy worked well when the EU's legitimacy had to be in the eyes of Member State governments, which had the technical expertise to see the advantages of EU structures and policies, including the ability to cast blame on the EU. It is harder to gain in the eyes of citizens.

Throughput legitimacy is the third kind of legitimacy that the EU seeks: emphasizing the legitimacy of its actions through extensive consultation, efforts at transparency and the cultivation of links with stakeholders including interest groups and civil society. It is perhaps most developed in the area of trade policy but it is a strategy deployed throughout EU governance.[51] Throughput legitimacy, in other words, amounts to the proposition that even if the EU lacks the input legitimacy that Member States enjoy, and even if Member State governments try to take the credit for successful policies and blame the EU for unpopular policies, its policy process legitimates the outcomes and builds legitimacy among groups in civil society and elsewhere who appreciate the opportunity to participate.

EU stakeholder politics and political process are distinctive because of a widespread assumption that it must develop its input and output legitimacy, and compensate for any failings with superior throughput legitimacy. In other words, lacking a clear *demos* and often making policies which are not very visible, understood and attractive, its governance relies particularly heavily on listening to stakeholders and even helping to create them when the existing interest group ecology of Brussels does not produce them. The result is an interest group environment that is fragmented and open to money, yet at the same time attentive to diverse interests that wield little political power.

2.3.2 Identifying stakeholders in Brussels

In other words, stakeholders in EU policy are very important, for assisting with throughput legitimacy and for helping policy-makers understand the complexities of a union with over 500 million people. Identifying key stakeholders interested in health in the European Union is not as easy as it may sound. Researchers have used a variety of techniques, but each has drawbacks born of a simple

---

51 Jarman H (2017). Trade policy governance: What health policymakers and advocates need to know. *Health Policy*, 121(11):1105–12.

problem: the EU makes it easy to engage at a very superficial level, but there are major time and resource constraints that mean the actual number of reliably engaged stakeholders who are seen as serious is much smaller. Time and resource constraints also mean that money is empowered, for it can buy staff time and capacity. In the particular context of the EU, throughput legitimacy also means that poorly resourced interests are often better positioned and supported to act in policy than their equivalents in Member States which are less concerned about throughput legitimacy.

One alternative option is to consult the various lists of organizations that respond to consultations, join consultative forums, appear in lobbying directories sold around Brussels, and send representatives to public meetings. This produces a long list of organizations. The EU Health Policy Forum has around 5000 registered organizations and it is not easy to find out what they are (EU stakeholder transparency initiatives have a strange way of making such information less accessible and transparent with each initiative). We can take it as a given that they are not all equally influential in policy debates. Statistical research, albeit rather old, has indeed found that most of the organizations that appear as interested in EU health policy are not really very interested and are not very influential.[52] In many cases, especially with local and regional governments and Member State level associations, the main function of the office in Brussels is to watch for funding opportunities and take note of consequential policies rather than lobby. In particular, the EU has an institutional bias towards interacting with "Eurogroups", EU-level associations, rather than organizations set up at Member State level. The reliance on Eurogroups can appear to freeze out national expertise, but it has two compelling advantages: it obliges Eurogroups, rather than the Commission, to aggregate diverse preferences, and it obliges stakeholders to formulate broad appeals rather than speak in the particularistic languages of national politics and special interests.

The main alternative is to ask practitioners which the key organizations are. This method has several drawbacks. One is that it risks mapping networks rather than the whole field: if you start by asking public health advocates, you will end with a better map of public health advocates than of, for example, anti-deregulation advocates employed by industry. The second is that the field of health policy is essentially contested – are manufacturers of sugary industrial sweets part of the health policy world, in their own eyes or in the eyes of others? They are certainly to be found in the Health Policy Forum and other consultative bodies. The third is that Brussels, like any heavily lobbied political system, has lobbying firms with the capacity to rapidly expand their operations at every level, from junior to senior,

---

52   Greer SL, Massard da Fonseca E, Adolph C (2008). Mobilizing Bias in Europe: Lobbies, Democracy and EU Health Policy-Making. *European Union Politics*, 9(3):403–33.

when an industry with money finds that an issue is on the agenda and wants to influence it. Temporary lobbying operations of great size can be set up almost overnight if there is enough money. Fourth and finally, lobbying can be murky. Not all organizations like to represent themselves publicly as such. Industries with serious opposition in the health world, notably the tobacco industry, frequently have incentives to work through other organizations, funding and supporting groups whose link to the underlying industry support is not made clear.

There are some clear repeat players in EU health policy with credibility and a health agenda, such as the European Public Health Alliance (EPHA) made up of public health NGOs, the more academic European Public Health Association (EUPHA), the European Trades Union Institute, the European Consumer Organization (BEUC), the European Patients Forum, the European Heart Network, the Association International de la Mutualité (AIM) and European Social Insurance Platform, representing social insurance organizations and associations for various health professions, to name just a few. Many 'non health' NGOs now occupy key positions in health-related discussions such as transport (TE – Transport Environment), housing/homeless (FEANTSA – European Federation of National Organisations Working with the Homeless)[53] and environment (HEAL – European Health and Environment Alliance) to name but a few. There are also Member State level organizations that have credibility even if they must often formally act through Eurogroups.[54]

In most cases, the size of these organizations' staff is very small and the number of their senior or long-term staff smaller still. This means that their credibility and profile in Brussels can rise and fall quickly with internal politics and the career choices of individuals – while it is easy to staff these organizations at the junior level, thanks to the large Brussels labour market in public affairs staff, it is relatively hard to find or train people who will develop technical and political

---

53 Homelessness, particularly chronic homelessness, often reflects health problems, and being homeless is extremely bad for one's health. Willison C (2017). Shelter from the Storm: Roles, responsibilities, and challenges in United States housing policy governance. *Health Policy*, 121(11):1113–23. For European data, and EU policy options, see FEANTSA and the Fondation Abbé Pierre (2019). Fourth Overview of Housing Exclusion in Europe 2019. Available at: https://www.feantsa.org/en/report/2019/04/01/the-fourth-overview-of-housing-exclusion-in-europe-2019?bcParent=27. Brussels: FEANTSA; Clair A, Stuckler D (2016). Structured Review of the Evidence on the Intersection of Housing and Health Policy in the WHO European Region. *Public Health Panorama*, 2(2):160–83.

54 For more information and research about EU stakeholder engagement, there are a number of useful texts: Woll C (2008). *Firm Interests: How Governments Shape Business Lobbying on Global Trade*. Ithaca: Cornell University Press; Greer SL (2009). "The Changing World of European Health Lobbies", in Coen C & Richardson JJ (eds.). *Lobbying in the European Union*. Oxford: Oxford University Press; Coen D (ed.) (2007). EU Lobbying: Empirical and Theoretical Studies. Abingdon: Routledge; Greer SL, Massard da Fonseca E, Adolph C (2008). Mobilizing Bias in Europe: Lobbies, Democracy and EU Health Policy-Making. *European Union Politics*, 9(3):403–33; van Schendelen MP, Van Schendelen R (2010). *More Machiavelli in Brussels: The art of lobbying the EU*. Amsterdam University Press. Some of these titles may seem old, but, while specific information about EU politics and people changes daily, the basics of EU stakeholder engagement and the world of interest representation change much more slowly.

credibility over years. Many of the most effective organizations are precisely the ones which have been able to retain staff for years, keep in touch with "alumni" who have moved on, and develop strong cadres of junior and mid-level staff. Succession and workforce planning are therefore crucial in these organizations, and for outside observers it is important to pay attention to individual people's careers as well as their organizations.

2.3.3   Forums, platforms, consultations and meetings

Throughout this book there will be references to a variety of forums, platforms and consultations. These are different ways in which the EU attempts to gain information, perspective and throughput legitimacy for its actions.

Consultations are mandatory (Box 2.1) as part of the proposal process and solicit views on proposed legislation (the EP, the Council and other EU institutions view themselves as having legitimacy by election and do not consult, though they can and do make many kinds of inquiries). Most consultations receive relatively few responses, though a few have been "flooded" by organized interests (*see* section 3.1.1).

The Commission, including DG SANTE, has also worked through a large number of forums, notably the Health Policy Forum, platforms and regular meetings. Their goals range from seeking information to educating participants to making commitments to policy actions. They are discussed throughout chapter 3, especially in 3.1 (for public health initiatives) and 3.6 (for health policy and health systems initiatives).

2.3.4   Supporting stakeholders: money, media, industry and civil society

"Follow the money" is always good advice. In the relatively open and fragmented world of EU interest groups, it is particularly good advice. It leads to both attentiveness to lobbying strategies that might not be obvious, such as sponsoring events with no clear lobbying content in order to build credibility, and to the ways in which the Commission, seeking information and throughput legitimacy, has historically sought to provide resources to civil society organizations that can break what might otherwise be a steady diet of industry-funded lobbying.

One of the key issues in any area of EU policy is the extent of Commission support for civil society organizations. A basic fact of interest representation in Brussels, as in most political systems, is that business organizations far outnumber and are far better resourced than other parts of society. Throughput legitimacy (*see* section 2.2), as well as informed policy, requires broader participation than industry lobbies will ever provide.[55] The Commission, in any policy field, thus supports Eurogroups and others to connect with broader social interests and represent views from those sectors.[56]

There are a number of structural threats to this arrangement. One is that Brussels organizations become more focused on getting and keeping Commission funding, which can often come through distorting programmes, than on serving their members. Maintaining responsiveness and accountability to complex membership bases with different understandings of the EU is a structural problem for any Eurogroup. Another is that the political leadership of the EU might decide that it can do with less throughput legitimacy and civil society information, and reduce the funding for civil society. Political leaders can also pick and choose the organizations they fund, shaping the civil society they want to hear from. If the political leadership of the EU feels confident in its input or output legitimacy, then it might not see the case for subsidizing those with contrary views. Even if there is no such preference, the end of the Health Programme and occasional poor connections between CHAFEA (*see* section 2.1.6) and the Commission policy staff can lead to funding decisions not always aligning with the need for strong and diverse voices in Brussels health politics.

Beyond the visible and formal world of advocates and lobbies in Brussels, there are other ways that moneyed interests can influence policy. "Think tanks" of various sorts regularly appear in Brussels with background interests and funding that are unclear. Even long-established think tanks with some credibility will often have funders who shape their agendas and policy interests. Industries that know they are divisive will frequently have the most incentive to act through think tanks and public affairs consultants, but almost any interest can be found doing it. Civil servants and academics face reputational and professional risks in being seen as advocates or lobbyists, but it is wise to assume that anybody involved in politics is explicitly involved in advocating for a position, and is being held accountable for their effectiveness at it.

Finally, Brussels media suffers from a particularly severe version of the problems affecting media across Europe. Not only is it difficult to find a business model today that will sustain expert and investigative journalism, but the EU media sphere is fragmented, the audience for EU politics is small and specific, and EU activities are often technical and of interest to small groups. The result is a variety

---

55   Schmidt VA (2013). Democracy and legitimacy in the European Union revisited: Input, output and 'throughput'. *Political Studies*, 61(1):2–22; Greer SL et al. (2017). *Civil society and health: contributions and potential*. Copenhagen: WHO Regional office for Europe, on behalf of the European Observatory on Health Systems and Policies.

56   Passarani I (2017). "Engaging with civil society: the successful example of the European Medicines Agency", in Greer SL et al. (2017). *Civil society and health: contributions and potential*. Copenhagen: WHO Regional office for Europe, on behalf of the European Observatory on Health Systems and Policies, pp. 67–82.

of media at work: elite global press with strong EU coverage but their own biases, clear points of view and lack of interest in most EU dossiers (e.g. the *Financial Times, Economist, Le Monde*); EU-focused generalist press whose business model makes them prone to dependence on advertising and sponsorship from interest groups (e.g. Euractiv, Politico.eu[57]); and specialist industry press which focuses on the issues of interest to particular industries and is typically expensive and targeted at narrow, business, audiences. Surrounding this media is a blizzard of newsletters and policy reports of varying quality from trade associations, law firms, consultants, lobbyists and others, of often unknown motivations, who view production of news as a useful way to shape agendas and thinking. It is no wonder that it is even harder to navigate this landscape than it is to work out what is happening in Member State capitals or that so many groups decide the solution is to employ Brussels staff just to figure out what is going on.

2.4   Agendas and the Sustainable Development Goals in the EU[58]

From the Single Europe Act, with its ambition of internal market unification by 1992, to the Lisbon Agenda, the EU has adopted overarching goals. For the first time it has adopted global goals as the replacement for its Europe 2020 agenda: the Sustainable Development Goals (SDGs). Just as the SEA or Lisbon Agenda or Europe 2020 authorized action and policy development, the SDGs authorize thinking and even action on a broad range of globally important issues. In her speech to the European Parliament before it voted on her appointment as President of the European Commission, Ursula von der Leyen announced that she would "refocus our European Semester to make sure that we stay on track with our Sustainable Development Goals".[59]

The SDGs are the 17 goals, with 169 discrete targets, agreed by the United Nations (Box 2.6) in 2015 as part of its Agenda 2030 programme. They are the successors to the Millennium Development Goals but, unlike the MDGs, they go

---

57   politico.eu, for example, has run multiple timely stories about tobacco politics but is also, in 2019, being investigated by Belgian authorities on the suspicion that its partnership with British American Tobacco violates tobacco advertising law. Even if BAT somehow did not influence coverage or choice of topics, the partnership nevertheless "normalizes" the tobacco industry as a legitimate part of politics, contrary to tobacco control advocates' powerful strategy of denormalizing the industry. *See* Peter Teffer, "Belgium prepares probe into Politico tobacco sponsorship", *EU Observer*, 27 June 2019. Available at: https://euobserver.com/health/145285. For denormalization, see Jarman H (2019). Normalizing Tobacco? The Politics of Trade, Investment, and Tobacco Control. *The Milbank Quarterly*, 97(2):449–79.

58   The lead author for this section was Tugce Schmitt.

59   European Commission (2019). Opening Statement in the European Parliament Plenary Session by Ursula von der Leyen, Candidate for President of the European Commission, Strasbourg, 16 July 2019. Available at: http://europa.eu/rapid/press-release_SPEECH-19-4230_en.htm.

Box 2.6   *Sustainable Development Goals in the EU*

The European Union has committed to implement the following SDGs in both its internal and its external policies:

1. To end poverty in all its forms everywhere.
2. To end hunger, achieve food security and improved nutrition, and promote sustainable agriculture
3. To ensure healthy lives and promote well-being for all at all ages
4. To ensure inclusive and equitable quality education and promote life-long learning opportunities for all
5. To achieve gender equality and empower all women and girls
6. To ensure availability and sustainable management of water and sanitation for all
7. To ensure access to affordable, reliable, sustainable and modern energy for all
8. To promote sustained, inclusive and sustainable economic growth, full and productive employment and decent work for all
9. To build resilient infrastructure, promote inclusive and sustainable industrialization and foster innovation
10. To reduce inequality within and among countries
11. To make cities and human settlements inclusive, safe, resilient and sustainable
12. To ensure sustainable consumption and production patterns
13. To take urgent action to combat climate change and its impacts
14. To conserve and sustainably use oceans, seas and marine resources for sustainable development
15. To protect, restore and promote sustainable use of terrestrial ecosystems, sustainably manage forests, combat desertification, and halt and reverse land degradation and halt biodiversity loss
16. To achieve peaceful and inclusive societies, rule of law, effective and capable institutions
17. To strengthen means of implementation and revitalize the global partnership for sustainable development

---

far beyond development policy. A 2016 Commission Communication[60] adopted them as broader unifying goals for the EU. According to the 2016 "Key European action supporting the 2030 Agenda and the Sustainable Development Goals", the Commission has confirmed its commitment to sustainable development and its

---

60 COM(2016) 739 final. Communication from the Commission to the European Parliament, the Council, the European Economic and Social Committee and the Committee of the Regions. Next steps for a sustainable European future. European action for sustainability.

intention to further mainstreaming it into its policy-making.[61] In line with the principle of subsidiarity, the key European actions supporting the 2030 Agenda and the SDGs that would affect Member States differ from one SDG field to another. Depending on the SDG and its main policy fields, the EU is committed to putting a framework in place/supporting and complementing/ promoting the achievement of particular SDGs within the EU. There is a detailed EU policy action overview for each SDG. In the case of health, the obvious focus is SDG 3, which is a commitment "to ensure healthy lives and promote well-being for all at all ages". This includes universal health coverage as well as attention to the many determinants of health that the EU can affect.

A Multi-Stakeholder Platform was commissioned to report on ways the EU budget can support the SDGs.[62]

In October 2018 the European Council welcomed the intention of the Commission to publish a Reflection Paper to pave the way for a comprehensive implementation strategy in 2019. This paper puts forward three different scenarios following the European Council's guidance to lead the discussion on how the implementation of the SDGs could best be achieved and what would be the most effective division of roles. Three scenarios of the Commission as well as their advantages and disadvantages are published in this document (pp. 34–9), proposing different enforcement levels of the Commission on the MS.

Eurostat has since 2017 published a review of progress towards the SDG goals within the EU that builds on its SDG indicator set.[63] The reviews are instructive, reminding us that much needs to be done in rich countries as well as in poorer ones, in particular to achieve goals such as "Sustainable Consumption and Production" and even in areas where the EU is ahead of other rich polities, such as "sustainable cities and communities" and "climate action".

---

61 SWD(2016) 390 final. Commission Staff Working Document. Key European action supporting the 2030 Agenda and the Sustainable Development Goals. Accompanying the document, Communication from the Commission to the European Parliament, the Council, the European Economic and Social Committee and the Committee of the Regions. Next steps for a sustainable European future: European Union action for sustainability (COM(2016) 739 final), p. 2.

62 Implementing the Sustainable Development Goals through the next Multi-annual Financial Framework of the European Union (Advisory report to the European Commission by the Multi-Stakeholder Platform on the Implementation of the Sustainable Development Goals in the EU, March 2018). More information about the Multi-Stakeholder Platform can be found here: https://ec.europa.eu/info/strategy/international-strategies/eu-and-sustainable-development-goals/multi-stakeholder-platform-sdgs/role-structure-and-working-methods_en.

63 Eurostat, European Commission (2018). Sustainable development in the European Union: Monitoring report on progress towards the SDGs in an EU context. Publications Office of the European Union. A list of the platform members can be found at: https://ec.europa.eu/info/strategy/international-strategies/eu-and-sustainable-development-goals/multi-stakeholder-platform-sdgs/platform-members_en. Members of the Management Committee of the platform can be downloaded at: https://ec.europa.eu/info/files/members-management-committee-multi-stakeholder-platform-sustainable-development-goals_en.

In terms of their potential for health, most if not all of the SDGs have clear co-benefits: they are unlikely to be achieved without investment in health and health systems, and they are likely to have benefits for health and health systems. Exploring co-benefits is a way to give some coherence to intersectoral conversations and authorize advocates to push for these objectives in the face of bureaucratic, political and other pressures to de-emphasize these goals and the broad policy work needed to achieve them.

2.5   Conclusion

The particular institutional structure and history of the EU has given it a distinctive, and often powerful, set of policies for health. The institutional structures here help to explain how it has been created and how it might change, and help to identify some of the levers and options within the system. They show, in part, how legal bases are crucial but do not always determine what happens. Environmental policy in the EU was improving health from at least 1975 under internal market treaty bases, but environmental policy only appeared in the treaties in 1992, at the same time as public health. The difference was not in the treaties; it was in the willingness of the EU's leadership to use internal market policies to make environmental law.

The next three chapters discuss the three faces of the EU health policies that have emerged from the interplay of institutions, legal bases and politics. The first is explicit policies for health. The second face is internal market policies that affect health, from medicines regulation to competition law. The third face, finally, is fiscal governance. Each works in quite different ways but all three can contribute to health.

Chapter 3

EU action for health

The first face of EU health policy is the most obvious: actions to improve health. There is a treaty article (168) called public health, a directorate-general for health (called SANTE) and a set of health forums, strategies and plans. It is a site of institutional creativity because subsidiarity is taken particularly seriously by health ministers and Member States who are reluctant to see EU policy affect healthcare systems. As a result, its effects are often powerful but hard to see – in shaping information, agendas, expectations and data itself, from case definitions in epidemiology to good practice in primary care.

3.1 Public health

Right from the introduction of a specific article on health in the Maastricht Treaty (formally the Treaty on European Union) in 1992,[1] the issue with EU powers on health has been striking a balance between potential common interests in working on health and the high degree of national sensitivity and specificity about health matters. This is reflected in the complex drafting of that article, in particular the requirement that the Union "respect the responsibilities of the Member States" for their health systems.[2] Although legally this provision does not really add much to the formal division of powers throughout the treaties, it highlights the concerns of national governments in drafting the treaty provisions on health.

The division of competences is summarized at the start of the TFEU, which came into force in 2009. The only area of shared competence between the EU and the Member States is "common safety concerns in public health matters";[3] for the wider objective of the "protection and improvement of human health"[4] the EU may only "support, coordinate or supplement" Member States' actions.[5]

The first point to note about the main article (TFEU Article 168, which appears in Box 1.4 and the Appendix) is that it is not an article on health, but an article on *public* health. This again is a deliberate attempt by the drafters of the treaties

---

1   European Communities (1992). *Treaty on the European Union.* Luxembourg: European Communities. Available at: http://www.eurotreaties.com/maastrichtec.pdf, accessed 1 May 2019 .
2   TFEU, Article 168, paragraph 7.
3   TFEU, Article 4, paragraph 2(k).
4   TFEU, Article 6, subparagraph (a).
5   TFEU, Article 6.

to orient EU action towards population-level measures and away from action on health services. The objective of restricting EU action in health care is reflected in the objectives of the Article, which are focused towards public health activities and health determinants (tobacco and alcohol being specifically mentioned).

The second point to note is that the powers given to the EU to achieve these public health objectives are very limited. The only area where binding legislation is called for covers concerns of quality and safety standards for substances of human origin, blood and blood derivatives.[6] Article 168 does also provide for the EU to provide financial support for actions more broadly in support of public health,[7] but this of course depends on the budgetary means available, which have in practice also been very limited. The article does include an "integration clause" requiring health protection to be ensured in all EU policies and activities,[8] but this does not in itself provide a basis for additional measures.

There are also some additional and unusual tools provided in Article 168. One is the power for the Council of Ministers to adopt recommendations in support of the objectives of the Article. These recommendations are non-binding legal acts. While these are not exactly the most powerful of instruments, they have been used to good effect in the health area, such as establishing a European commitment to cancer screening.[9]

Another unusual power is the provision for Member States to coordinate their own policies on areas too sensitive for legislation or outside their scope, working through "the establishment of guidelines and indicators, the organization of exchange of best practice, and the preparation of the necessary elements for periodic monitoring and evaluation".[10] This type of non-legislative cooperation has been mostly applied in the social policy area; so far it has not been widely used in the health area.

3.1.1 Tobacco control

Tobacco is one of the largest causes of sickness and death in the world and remains the largest avoidable health risk for people living in the EU. Although smoking prevalence has decreased in many Member States in recent years, the disparity among states in levels of smoking remains large. Concerns have also been raised about the potential health effects of the increasing use of non-traditional tobacco products such as e-cigarettes.

---

6   TFEU, Article 168, paragraph 4.
7   TFEU, Article 168, paragraph 5: "incentive measures" refers to financing tools, not binding legislation.
8   TFEU, Article 168, paragraph 1; *see also* Article 9.
9   Council of the European Union (2003). Council recommendation 2003/878/EC on cancer screening. *Official Journal*, L 327/34.
10   TFEU, Article 168, paragraph 2.

Best practice tobacco control policies are defined internationally by the acronym MPOWER. States should Monitor tobacco use via integrated surveillance policies, Protect people from second-hand smoke, Offer cessation support, Warn the public about the dangers of smoking (e.g. via warning labels and advertising), Enforce bans on tobacco advertising, promotion and sponsorship, and Raise taxes on tobacco. The EU and its Member States have been successful in some of these areas but not others (*see* Table 3.1). In particular, implementation of restrictions on exposure to second-hand smoke remains patchy. And while the EU has the potential for further action to raise the price of tobacco products (e.g. via an EU-wide minimum excise tax), these actions face political obstacles.

The EU's first tobacco policy was actually in support of tobacco, with the Common Agricultural Policy providing subsidies to tobacco growers from 1970 onwards. Considering that starting point, the EU has greatly improved its contribution to tobacco control over time. From the 1980s onwards, EU policy-makers adopted a wide variety of tobacco control measures (summarized in Table 3.1) despite strong opposition from the tobacco industry. EU subsidies to tobacco farmers were phased out entirely by 2010. The EU has also played a significant role in supporting international efforts to coordinate tobacco control policies across borders, primarily through the only international agreement against tobacco, the Framework Convention on Tobacco Control (FCTC).

The core of current tobacco regulation in the EU is the Tobacco Products Directive (TPD) (2014/40/EU). The TPD broadened the scope of EU tobacco regulation in some significant ways, including setting maximum permissible levels of tar, nicotine and carbon monoxide for cigarettes and establishing a framework to allow monitoring of further ingredients and emissions. The TPD requires Member States to ban tobacco products with certain additives, including those with a characterizing flavour (e.g. fruit, vanilla or menthol), those that ease inhalation (e.g. menthol or clove) or those with additives that have been proven to increase addiction (based on recent scientific studies, this category could also include menthol). The requirement to ban menthol products comes into effect in 2020.

In terms of warning the public about the dangers of tobacco products, the TPD requires that combined health warnings consisting of text plus a colour image must cover 65% of the front and back of tobacco packages (for smoking products only). Slim packages, which are often designed to resemble designer perfume packaging in order to appeal to women, are banned, as are misleading elements that make health claims about tobacco products, such as "free from additives". Cigarette packages must contain at least 20 cigarettes. The TPD stops short of mandating plain packaging, which is recognized internationally as the best practice standard, but it does not preclude Member States from adopting

Table 3.1 *EU Member State performance against WHO tobacco control targets*

Member State	Adult Daily Smoking Prevalence 2015	Monitoring	Smoke-Free Policies	Cessation	Health Warnings	Mass Media	Advertising Bans	Taxation	Cigarettes Less Affordable Since 2008?
Austria	2	4	1	3	4	4	3	4	Yes
Belgium	2	4	..	3	4	3	3	4	Yes
Bulgaria	2	4	4	3	4	1	3	4	No change
Croatia	1	4	2	3	2	1	3	4	Yes
Cyprus	2	3	3	3	2	4	3	4	Yes
Czechia	2	4	2	3	4	1	3	4	Yes
Denmark	3	4	1	4	4	4	3	3	Yes
Estonia	2	4	1	4	4	4	3	4	Yes
Finland	3	4	1	3	4	..	3	4	Yes
France	2	4	..	3	4	..	3	4	Yes
Germany	2	4	1	3	4	3	3	3	Yes
Greece	1	4	4	3	4	1	3	4	Yes
Hungary	2	4	3	3	4	1	3	3	Yes
Ireland	3	4	4	4	4	4	3	4	No change
Italy	2	4	..	3	4	4	3	4	Yes
Latvia	1	4	3	3	4	3	3	4	No change
Lithuania	2	4	2	3	4	1	3	4	No change
Luxembourg	3	4	1	4	2	..	3	3	Yes
Malta	2	4	4	4	4	4	3	4	No change
Netherlands	2	4	1	4	4	4	3	3	Yes
Poland	2	4	2	3	4	3	3	4	Yes
Portugal	3	4	3	3	4	4	3	3	Yes
Romania	2	4	4	3	4	3	3	3	Yes
Slovakia	2	4	2	3	4	1	3	4	Yes
Slovenia	3	4	..	3	2	1	3	4	Yes
Spain	2	4	4	3	3	1	4	4	Yes
Sweden	4	4	1	3	4	1	3	3	Yes
United Kingdom	3	4	4	4	4	4	3	4	Yes

Worst performance against WHO standards > ▨1 ▦2 ▩3 ■4 < Best performance against WHO standards

Source: WHO Report on the Global Tobacco Epidemic, 2017. More comprehensive analysis is available at https://www.who.int/tobacco/global_report/2017/en/

Table 3.2   *Summary of EU tobacco control legislation*

Name (year) of measure	Number	Key requirements
Labelling directives (1989, 1992)	89/622/EEC	Requires rotating health warnings on tobacco products
	92/41/EEC	Ban on the marketing of certain tobacco products for oral use
Advertising directives (1989, 1997, 1998, 2003)	89/552/EEC 97/36/EC	Ban all forms of TV advertising for tobacco products
	98/43/EC	Ban on tobacco advertising in the press, radio and on the Internet
	2003/33/EC	Ban on tobacco sponsorship of events with cross-border effects
Tar Yield Directive (1990)	90/239/EEC	Sets a maximum tar yield of 15mg per cigarette by 31 December 1992 and of 12mg per cigarette from 31 December 1997
Tax directives (1992, 1995, 2002, 2011)	92/78/EEC 92/79/EEC 92/80/EEC 95/59/EC 2002/10/EC 2011/64/EU	Set minimum levels of excise duties on cigarettes and tobacco
Tobacco Product Regulation Directive (2001)	2001/37/EC	Larger warning labels are required on all tobacco products; descriptors suggesting that one tobacco product is less harmful than another are banned; manufacturers and importers must submit a list of all ingredients used in the manufacture of tobacco products; maximum levels of tar, nicotine and carbon monoxide established for cigarettes (10mg tar, 1mg nicotine and 10mg carbon monoxide per cigarette)
Workplace Air Quality directives (1989, 1992)	89/654/EEC 92/57/EEC 92/91/EEC 92/104/EEC	Require employers to ensure that workers have access to fresh air and ventilation
Framework Directive on Health and Safety in the Workplace (1989)	89/391/EEC	Requires a health assessment to be carried out by employers, which should include exposure to second-hand smoke in the workplace
Asbestos Directive (1983)	83/477/EEC	Prohibits smoking in areas where asbestos is handled
Resolution on Smoking in Public Places (1989), Smoke-free Environments Recommendation (2009)		Invites Member States to adopt measures protecting people from exposure to smoke in indoor workplaces, public places and public transport
Pregnant Women Directive (1992)	92/85/EEC	Requires employers to take action to protect pregnant and breastfeeding women from exposure to an extensive list of substances, including carbon monoxide
Carcinogens Directive (1990)	90/394/EEC	Restricts smoking in workplace areas where carcinogenic substances are handled
Council Resolutions and Proposals to Member States and the Commission (1993, 1996, 1999) on measures to combat smoking (non-binding)		Various measures to combat smoking

Name (year) of measure	Number	Key requirements
Council recommendation (2003)	2003/54/EC	Concerns aspects of tobacco control that are the responsibility of the Member States, including tobacco sales to children and adolescents; tobacco advertising and promotion that has no cross-border effects; provision of information on advertising expenditure; environmental effects of tobacco smoke
WHO Framework Convention on Tobacco Control (2004)	2004/513/EC (Council adoption decision)	Wide-ranging global treaty on tobacco control
Tobacco Products Directive (2014)	2014/14/EU	Major legislation on tobacco products (see text)

Sources: Authors; ASPECT (Analysis of the Science and Policy for European Control of Tobacco) Consortium, *Tobacco or health in the European Union: past, present and future* (Luxembourg: Publications Office of the European Union, 2004; DG Health and Consumers, *Tobacco*. Available at: http://ec.europa.eu/health/tobacco/key_documents/index_en.htm#anchor1, accessed 14 July 2014)

more stringent packaging requirements. Subsequently a number of EU Member States have adopted plain packaging laws.

The TPD illustrates the high level of political controversy surrounding tobacco control policies in the EU. The legislation took five years to pass and two more to implement, during which time it was subject to intense lobbying by the tobacco industry, followed by several legal challenges. The initial introduction of the Directive was significantly delayed because of the sheer volume of response to the public consultation, leading some public health advocates to raise concerns that the tobacco industry was attempting to "flood" the consultation in order to buy time. The process was further disrupted by the abrupt departure of Commissioner Dalli, who was accused of holding off-the-record meetings with tobacco industry lobbyists – an activity that goes against the EU's stated position under the FCTC Article 5.3 guidelines that policy-makers should not have contact with the tobacco industry.

EU tobacco control policies have also been the subject of multiple legal challenges. The limitations of using the internal market treaty provisions as a basis for public health laws were illustrated clearly with the annulment of the first tobacco advertising directive by the European Court of Justice. This directive was also based on internal market provisions of the treaty but, following legal action brought by Germany, the Court annulled the directive on the grounds that the ban introduced by the directive went beyond what could be justified in order to enable functioning of the internal market, in particular for local products (e.g. parasols and other articles used in hotels).

This decision has proved to be an outlier, however. The Court did explicitly recognize the legitimacy of integrating health objectives alongside internal market objectives in principle. And the Court later upheld the second, narrower, directive on tobacco advertising when that was also contested by Germany on the grounds that its internal market legal base was not sufficient for its health effects.

In recent legal disputes relating to the TPD addressing product standardization, e-cigarettes, plain packaging, menthol and snus, the Court has emphasized health and the internal market as parallel functions of the EU, as well as emphasizing the EU's binding international commitments to adopt tobacco control policies under the FCTC.[11] Despite the TPD surviving each of these disputes, policy-makers should expect new tobacco control policies to be subject to challenges in the EU court system. Legislating and regulating in a way that makes it easier to defend against such suits, and then defending against them, will require extensive preparation and resources, strong adherence to governance procedures and accurate synthesis of large bodies of scientific evidence.[12]

Along these lines, a significant current and future challenge for the EU lies in the increasing diversity of tobacco products on the market. While a large body of scientific evidence shows that traditional tobacco products such as cigarettes and cigars are extremely harmful for health, we know less about the long-term health risks of newer tobacco products such as e-cigarettes.

There are three main challenges for the EU in this regard: first, it can be challenging for policy-makers to reconcile different levels of scientific knowledge about different types of tobacco product with consistent public health messages. Second, differences between national approaches to newer tobacco products may have a deleterious effect on policy-making at the EU level. And third, keeping up with the diversity of the market requires considerable governance capacity.

The EU has already confronted this dilemma in seeking to regulate oral tobacco (defined as snus and moist snuff), where an exclusionary solution was reached – the sale of snus is banned in all EU countries except Sweden. Similar flexibilities are built into the TPD regarding the "characterizing flavours" ban, which does not apply at all to oral tobacco products. Member States can also decide to exempt other products from the Directive (e.g. cigarillos, pipe tobacco). The TPD regulates electronic cigarettes, categorizing them as consumer goods, and stipulates various product characteristics such as the maximum permissible concentration of nicotine. But the tobacco market evolves quickly, with new products (e.g. heat-not-burn) entering the market before any scientific evidence of potential long-term harm emerges to balance out industry-funded studies. It remains to be seen to what extent the EU can continue to build a political and legal consensus in favour of a strong and coordinated set of tobacco control policies.

---

11   Judgments of 4 May 2016, Pillbox 38 (C-477/14), Poland (C-358/14), Philip Morris Brands and others (C-547/14); Judgment of 22 November 2018, Swedish Match (C-151/17).

12   Jarman H (2014). *The politics of trade and tobacco control.* Palgrave Macmillan.

3.1.2   Diet, nutrition and physical activity

Noncommunicable diseases are a major health threat in the European Union, and at the root of many of them is some combination of poor diet (poor nutrition, sometimes food poverty), obesity and a lack of exercise.[13] The European Union's contribution to the prevention of noncommunicable diseases is multiple and ambiguous: food safety, infrastructure investment, protected designation of origin law,[14] European Semester advice, climate change policy, trade policy and agricultural policy all affect diet, nutrition and physical activity for better or for worse. There is scope for a great deal of policy coherence – or policy incoherence.[15]

"Diet, Nutrition and Physical Activity" came onto the EU agenda as such under the Barroso Commission, with a flurry of initiatives: a 2005 Green Paper and a 2005 Nutrition Strategy White Paper,[16] and Health Programme initiatives as well as the innovative Platform on Diet, Nutrition and Physical Activity. The initiative was enterprising but was led by DG SANCO in an environment in which restrictive legislation on the topic was hard to imagine. As a result, it was creative but it left largely untouched important EU tools in areas such as agricultural policy and infrastructure. Instead, the strategy focused on a collaborative approach of looking for win-win solutions. The Platform brought together different kinds of organization, from Member States to industry to NGOs. It informed them of Commission thinking and they informed the Commission of their thinking, but the Platform's hope and promise were located in a system of commitments in which members would make commitments to improve diet, nutrition or physical activity (e.g. improving the nutritional quality of a food by a specified amount).

It was easy to criticize the Platform since participants made their own commitments; some NGOs saw it as a way for industry to pre-empt real regulation and make itself look good but nonetheless continued to participate because it was a structured way to engage with the Commission. That said, there are two conditions under which industry self-regulation is likely to work, and the EU is not as far from them as some Member States are. One condition for self-regulation

---

13 As many have noted, if exercise were a pill, it would be hailed as a miracle drug and widely prescribed. That raises the question of why so many aspects of our lives seem designed to prevent it, from buildings without visible and accessible stairs to roads that make it difficult to walk or ride a bicycle. For a particularly well presented discussion of the medical benefits of exercise, *see Exercise – The Miracle Cure*. London: Academy of Medical Royal Colleges, 2015. Available at: https://www.aomrc.org.uk/reports-guidance/exercise-the-miracle-cure-0215/.

14 The European legal framework for the protection of certain foods from particular places, produced in certain ways, e.g. the French *Appellation d'origine contrôlée* designation.

15 For example, Parsons K, Hawkes C (2018). *Connecting food systems for co-benefits: How can food systems combine diet-related health with environmental and economic policy goals?* Policy Brief. Copenhagen: WHO Regional office for Europe, on behalf of the European Observatory on Health Systems and Policies. Available at: http://www.euro.who.int/__data/assets/pdf_file/0007/387070/policy-brief-31-austria-eng.pdf.

16 COM(2007) 279 final. White Paper on a Strategy for Europe on Nutrition, Overweight and Obesity-related health issues.

is the threat of regulation – the explicit or implicit threat that if the industry does not improve its behaviour, policy-makers will force it to. That condition has been absent from EU food policy for some years and the senescence of these initiatives reflects that. The other condition is predictability. If industry is confident that any given policy initiative will end with the departure of the sponsoring minister, then it will have little incentive to change. If a stable institutional and legal structure gives industry incentive to act in a trustworthy manner and encourages longer-term reciprocity, then self-regulation and public-private initiatives can work.[17] The EU's very rigidity, born of its complex lawmaking procedure, makes it relatively predictable and therefore a potentially hospitable environment for effective self-regulation.

The topic may continue to loom large in Europe's public health challenges, in informed public health thinking, and in the minds of the many who are trying to eat and live better, but it has been sliding off the EU agenda since 2014. The Platform lost momentum when senior Commission officials ceased to attend; after a few meetings at which the Commission sent substitutes, most other organizations started to send junior staff as well. The political turn against regulation and in favour of growth in Europe reduced the threat of legislation and regulation that makes self-regulation effective, and the Platform, along with the similar Alcohol Forum, ceased to look relevant. In July 2019 civil society organizations focused on health (including BEUC, the European Heart Network and EPHA) walked out of the Platform, arguing that the "Platform, as it is currently constructed, is not fit for purpose and cannot therefore adequately contribute to reverse this tide. Indeed, the continual decreases in resources, time and attention afforded to the Platform over the years point to an acknowledgement of the limited impact that this forum, and the voluntary approach it embodies, can have."[18] This demarche was both predictable – the changing political scene constrained the possible relevance of such a Platform more every year since it was created – and means that there is a clear field for new policy and process thinking on food and public health in the new post-2019 EU.

3.1.3 Alcohol

Alcohol is a particularly European determinant of health; Europe has the highest consumption of alcohol per head in the world (almost double the global

---

17 Bekker MP et al. (2018). Comparative institutional analysis for public health: governing voluntary collaborative agreements for public health in England and the Netherlands. *European Journal of Public Health*, 28(suppl3):19–25.

18 Brussels, 3 July 2019, Civil Society Organisations Leave the EU Platform for Diet, Physical Activity and Health: https://epha.org/wp-content/uploads/2019/07/joint-statement-leaving-eu-diet-and-physical-activity-platform-july2019.pdf.

average),[19] although there has been an overall but uneven decline in (recorded) alcohol consumption since the early 1990s. Although alcohol is considered to be the third largest risk factor for ill-health in the EU,[20] it is also a major part of European society. Quite apart from its economic contribution (e.g. the EU produces more than half of the world's wine[21]), alcohol in its various forms is a central part of European culture and politics.[22] The EU's now-expired strategy regarding alcohol and health was, therefore, much more nuanced and limited than that for tobacco, focusing on education and discouraging drinking among particular groups, notably children, pregnant women and people driving cars – the populations and actions on which the industry already said it agreed.[23] The means used are also much softer than for tobacco, with the EU pursuing this strategy through supporting guidelines, exchanges of good practice, research and monitoring, rather than with legislation (although of course there is also relevant legislation, in particular the EU requirement that all alcoholic drinks show the strength of alcohol on their label[24]). On the face of it, this might seem a little weak; if alcohol is such a major determinant, why is the action to address it so limited, particularly in comparison to tobacco?

One obvious answer is that there is a broad social consensus on combating tobacco across Europe that does not exist for alcohol, which clearly affects the feasibility of Europe-wide measures. The well-established and well-known differences in national traditions regarding alcohol have made it difficult to establish the basics of a policy discussion about alcohol as a social determinant of health. This is changing, however, in part because of European integration and the growth of very large international companies that have worked out how to homogenize products in Europe with new products such as alcopops. Policy-makers who defend traditional alcohol use and regulatory patterns sometimes rethink in the face of such homogenizing of new products.[25] Moreover, the relationship between public policy and alcohol consumption is not straightforward. The

19 WHO Regional Office for Europe (2013). *Status report on alcohol and health in 35 European countries 2013*. Copenhagen: WHO Regional Office for Europe.
20 DG Health and Consumer Protection (2009). *First progress report on the implementation of the EU alcohol strategy*. Brussels: European Commission.
21 European Commission (2014). *What is the current situation of the European Union's wine sector?* Brussels: European Commission. Available at: http://ec.europa.eu/agriculture/markets/wine/index_en.htm, accessed 4 July 2014.
22 Colman T (2008). *Wine politics: How governments, environmentalists, mobsters, and critics influence the wines we drink*. University of California Press.
23 European Commission (2006). *An EU strategy to support Member States in reducing alcohol related harm (COM(2006)625)*. Brussels: European Commission.
24 European Commission (1987). Directive 87/250/EEC on the indication of alcoholic strength by volume in the labelling of alcoholic beverages for sale to the ultimate consumer. *Official Journal*, L 113/57.
25 Cisneros Ornberg J (2013). "Alcohol policy in the European Union", in Greer SL & Kurzer P (eds). *European Union public health policies: regional and global perspectives*. Abingdon: Routledge, pp. 168–80.

AMPHORA (Alcohol Public Health Research Alliance) project[26] has brought together evidence on alcohol and policy across Europe; this shows that, while overall there is an impact from restrictive measures, these interact with wider social changes (such as urbanization or changes in working patterns) and informal social norms (which tend to be the opposite to formal policies, meaning that where social norms are restrictive, such as in southern Europe, formal policies are relatively liberal, and vice versa),[27] as well as the history of different countries.

Nevertheless, although the relationship is complex, the AMPHORA alliance concluded that the evidence shows more-restrictive alcohol policies do have an impact in reducing harm from alcohol. So could the EU do more to address this, using stronger tools than used so far? This can be considered for three key aspects of alcohol policies: physical availability, economic availability and advertising and labelling.

Regarding physical availability, a key example is the restrictive retail monopolies on alcohol sales in Sweden and Finland, which constitute a strong limitation on the physical availability of alcohol. These were challenged before the European Court of Justice on the basis that such a monopoly was contrary to the EU's internal market.[28] However, the Court did not agree, accepting the argument that the monopoly was an appropriate tool to protect public health. So while it has not been easy to extend alcohol regulation, the EU internal market has not prevented Member States from having such controls on physical availability at national level.[29]

For economic availability, the central tool is taxation; increasing the cost of the product reduces consumption. Conversely, the main impact of the internal market on increased alcohol consumption in Sweden and Finland has not come from any increases in physical availability but rather from the increased availability of alcohol at much lower prices because of lower rates of excise duty in neighbouring countries to the south.[30] This is not a consequence of a lack of powers for the EU to act, as there is already legislation on excise duties for alcohol.[31] However, unlike for tobacco, that legislation has not been used to set a high minimum

---

26 The AMPHORA (Alcohol Measures for Public Health Research Alliance) project [web site], 2012. Available at: http://amphoraproject.net, accessed 4 July 2014.

27 Anderson B, Reynolds G (eds.) (2012). *Making and implementing European alcohol policy*. The AMPHORA (Alcohol Measures for Public Health Research Alliance) project.

28 European Court of Justice. Case C-189/95 *Franzén*.

29 *See* the classic book, Kurzer P (2001). *Markets and moral regulation: cultural change in the European Union*. Cambridge: Cambridge University Press.

30 Tigerstedt C et al. (2006). "Health in alcohol policies: the European Union and its Nordic Member States", in Ståhl T et al. (eds.). *Health in all policies: prospects and potentials*. Helsinki: Ministry of Social Affairs and Health, pp. 111–28.

31 Council of the European Union (1992). *Directive 92/83/EEC on the harmonization of the structures of excise duties on alcohol and alcoholic beverages; Directive 92/84/EEC on the approximation of the rates of excise duty on alcohol and alcoholic beverages*. Luxembourg: Publications Office of the European Union.

level of excise duty and thus price for alcohol throughout Europe. One does not have to look far to understand why; unlike tobacco (production of which has been relatively limited in the EU and concentrated in a few countries), alcohol production is spread much more widely throughout the EU, and for taxation legislation such as this, the unanimous agreement of EU Member States in the Council is required. Even a Commission proposal[32] to at least upgrade the current minimum levels of excise duty on alcohol has failed to make progress in the Council and was rejected outright by the European Parliament. So while the legal capacity is there, the democratic agreement in the legislative bodies of the EU to price alcohol more highly seems to be lacking.

In fact, the EU's constitutional asymmetry has slowed efforts to reduce alcohol use through minimum price legislation.[33] Scotland introduced a minimum price for alcohol in its 2012 Alcohol (Minimum Pricing) Act. The alcohol industry, led by the Scotch Whisky Association,[34] argued that it was discriminatory under EU law, and a preliminary reference was filed. The CJEU ruled that minimum pricing was permissible under Article 36 TFEU, which is the Article allowing for public health exceptions to free trade within the EU. It ruled, however, that a proportionality test applies and should be carried out by Member State courts, which gives them considerable latitude.[35]

The story is similar for the advertising and labelling of alcohol. Given the existing restrictions on advertising and labelling of tobacco products, there is clearly legal scope for the EU to do much more in restricting advertising of alcoholic products and to label them more clearly. Culturally, however, the acceptance of risks from tobacco is entirely different from the perceived risks of alcohol – and while that might be considered in itself an argument for EU action, it also underlines the likely difficulties on reaching agreement on more-restrictive advertising or labelling rules.

Another tool to prevent or reduce the harm from alcohol is labelling. The Commission audited in 2013–2014 the use of health-related messages on alcoholic

---

32   European Commission (2006). *Proposal for a Council Directive amending Directive 92/84/EEC on the approximation of the rates of excise duty on alcohol and alcoholic beverages (COM(2006)486)*. Brussels: European Commission.

33   For the Scottish experience, see Katikireddi SV, Bond L, Hilton S (2014). Changing policy framing as a deliberate strategy for public health advocacy: a qualitative policy case study of minimum unit pricing of alcohol. *The Milbank Quarterly*, 92(2):250–83; Katikireddi SV et al. (2014). Understanding the development of minimum unit pricing of alcohol in Scotland: a qualitative study of the policy process. *PLoS One*, 9(3):e91185.

34   This association represents producers of single malt whiskies, which are always priced far above the minimum price. Those producers are, however, an important Scottish export industry, tourist attraction and famous part of Scottish heritage, so it was a political tactic to have them lead the litigation instead of the less prestigious alcohol producers and retailers (e.g. fortified wine and discounting supermarkets) that would actually be affected.

35   Rieder CM (2017). "Courts and EU Health Law and Policy", in Hervey T, Young C & Bishop L (eds.). *Research Handbook in EU Health Law and Policy*. Cheltenham: Edward Elgar Publishing, pp. 60–81.

beverage labels. The study aimed to address the lack of information on the extent to which alcohol labelling was implemented in that period.[36] The Commission found that fewer than one in five alcohol labels (17%) contained a health-related message in addition to the alcohol content information mandatory in each country. Wine labels most often carried health-related messages (19%), with messages less frequently found on spirits (15%) and beers (14%). The research also revealed wide divergence in the type and form of health-related messages on alcohol labelling across Europe and highlighted the need for more stringent legal requirements regarding health-related labels.

These policy proposals were resubmitted for considerations by EU institutions in 2017. On 13 March 2017 the Commission adopted a report to the European Parliament and the Council regarding the mandatory labelling of the list of ingredients and the nutrition declaration of alcoholic beverages.[37] On 12 March 2018 the alcoholic beverage industry submitted a self-regulatory proposal to the Commission, which is currently under review. As of 2019, no alcoholic beverage containing more than 1.2% alcohol by volume (abv) is allowed to bear health claims. At the national level some Member States have adopted more voluntarist measures on the matter, including France and Lithuania, where labels on alcoholic beverages are required to warn consumers about the potential health consequences of drinking while being pregnant, either with a pictogram or with a text.

The same effort that we saw in food policy (*see* section 3.1.4) to build consensus and seek positive-sum solutions, or at least keep an issue on the agenda when there would be no real regulation, explained the creation of the Alcohol and Health Forum. This was another stakeholder forum including industry as well as civil society. It started operation in 2009.[38] In 2015, representatives of 20 public health civil society organizations walked out. They included the European Public Health Alliance (EPHA), the Standing Committee of European Doctors (CPME), and Eurocare, a Eurogroup focused on preventing and treating alcohol abuse. Their departure was a protest against the failure of the Commission to produce a new strategy after the 2013 expiry of the previous one. Even if it did not prompt the Commission to develop a new strategy, it made it clear that the politics of 2015 were hostile to regulation of a powerful industry.

---

36 European Commission (2014). State of play in the use of alcoholic beverage labels to inform consumers about health aspects. Action to prevent and reduce harm from alcohol. Brussels: European Commission.

37 European Commission (2017). Report from the Commission to the European Parliament and the Council regarding the mandatory labelling of the list of ingredients and the nutrition declaration of alcoholic beverages. Brussels: European Commission.

38 Celia C, Diepeveen S, Ling T (2010). The European Alcohol and Health Forum: First Monitoring Progress Report. Santa Monica, CA: RAND Corporation. Available at: https://www.rand.org/pubs/technical_reports/TR779.html.

3.1.4 Food safety

While nobody can deny the importance of food safety and the closely linked area of veterinary health to overall human public health, food safety is generally seen as a world distinctive from the public health world.[39] That outlook obscures the scale, complexity, and ambition of what the EU has done to construct a distinctive food safety regime. Food safety, which along with public health, is the core of DG SANTE's responsibilities, is a broad area of impressive regulatory complexity stretching from agriculture to restaurants, involving a variety of organizations at every level, from "farm to table" in the language of the field. An EU fact sheet claims that it involves 100 000–120 000 staff with specific inspection competencies regarding 25 million operators along the agrifood chain, a very large regulatory apparatus and task.[40]

Food safety has been a major issue for the EU, since the close integration of the food chain and food sector has led to scandals, of which the most politically consequential was BSE.[41] While there is constant pressure to reduce regulatory burdens on affected industries, the history of cross-border food safety crises in the EU creates a countervailing constituency for EU action. Scandals, whether they concern contaminated sprouts in Germany or mislabeled horsemeat in Ireland, regularly recur, showing gaps in the system and diminishing the effectiveness of those who might urge deregulation.

A 2002 General Food Law Regulation[42] both set out a philosophy for food safety whose recitals are unusually readable and established the European Food Safety Authority, based in Helsinki.[43] Its treaty bases are diverse but in this case mutually reinforcing and powerful – the powers to establish a Common Agricultural Policy, to consolidate the internal market, to establish a Common Commercial Policy, and the element of the public health article which allows

---

39 Grant W (2012). Agricultural Policy, Food Policy, and Communicable Disease Policy. *Journal of Health Politics, Policy and Law*, 37(6):1031–48; Lang IG (2017). "Public health in European Union food law", in Hervey T, Young C & Bishop L (eds.). *Research Handbook on EU Health Law and Policy*. Cheltenham: Edward Elgar Publishing, pp. 398–428.

40 Web site: https://ec.europa.eu/food/sites/food/files/safety/docs/fs_infograph_from-farm-to-fork_en.pdf.

41 Ansell C (2006). *What's the beef?: the contested governance of European food safety*. MIT Press; Ansell C, Gingrich J (2007). "The United Kingdom's Response to the BSE Epidemic", in Gibbons D (ed.). *Communicable crises: Prevention, response, and recovery in the Global Arena*. Information Age Publishing, pp. 169–202; Caduff L, Bernauer T (2006). Managing risk and regulation in European food safety governance. *Review of Policy Research*, (1):153–68.

42 Regulation (EC) No. 178/2002 of the European Parliament and of the Council of 28 January 2002 laying down the general principles and requirements of food law, establishing the European Food Safety Authority and laying down procedures in matters of food safety.

43 After a well-publicized argument with Italy, whose then prime minister grounded his case for a seat in Italy on his view that Italian cuisine was superior. The allocation of agencies at the Laeken summit was a nice example of the politics of agency allocation discussed in section 2.1.6. *See* BBC News, 16 December 2001: Food row blocked key EU decisions. Available at: http://news.bbc.co.uk/1/hi/world/europe/1714264.stm.

regulation of veterinary and phytosanitary issues with an impact on health.[44] (Note that consumer protection is missing and the public health treaty base reference is circumscribed.)

There was a reform to the General food law in 2019. In 2017 the citizens' initiative "Ban [the herbicide] glyphosate and protect people and the environment from toxic pesticides"[45] bore fruit in increased transparency. The Commission decided that glyphosates are not a threat to health and the environment, but it did agree to the second part of the initiative, which calls for the scientific evaluation of pesticides for EU regulatory approval based only on published studies, which are commissioned by competent public authorities instead of the pesticide industry. The reform, passed in the summer of 2019, expands the transparency of the assessment system, including that used by EFSA, by reducing commercial secrecy (e.g. use of copyright to avoid making toxins data public).[46]

The EU's basic approach, which has shaped international perceptions of best practice, explicitly invokes the precautionary principle (Box 3.3).[47] It focuses on four main areas: food hygiene, animal health, plant health, and contaminants and residues. Note that it is a food safety regime, not one focused on nutrition. Safe food need not be nutritious or otherwise healthy. There is, in fact, a certain tension between the highest standards of food safety and some of the more artisanal production methods found in Europe.

The overall EU approach is to maintain the security of the food chain from farm to fork, which entails a focus on traceability at every step from the farm to the fork – through agriculture in all its complexity, transport, retailing and food service. This is an ambitious goal, which the EU arguably takes more seriously than almost any other food system (contrast the United States, where traceability is far more primitive due to the well-documented lobbying of the

---

44 In the Amsterdam-era treaty articles cited in the legislation, Article 37, establishing CAP; Article 95, the procedural article for implementing Article 14, which is general internal market development; Article 133 establishing a common commercial policy, and Article 152(4)(b), concerning public health.

45 Commission registration number: ECI(2017)000002. Date of registration: 25 January 2017. "We call on the European Commission to propose to Member States a ban on glyphosate, to reform the pesticide approval procedure, and to set EU-wide mandatory reduction targets for pesticide use." Available at: https://ec.europa.eu/citizens-initiative/public/initiatives/successful/details/2017/000002?lg=en.

46 Council of the European Union. Proposal for a Regulation of the European Parliament and of the Council on the transparency and sustainability of the EU risk assessment in the food chain amending Regulation (EC) No. 178/2002 [on general food law], Directive 2001/18/EC [on the deliberate release into the environment of GMOs], Regulation (EC) No. 1829/2003 [on GM food and feed], Regulation (EC) No. 1831/2003 [on feed additives], Regulation (EC) No. 2065/2003 [on smoke flavourings], Regulation (EC) No. 1935/2004 [on food contact materials], Regulation (EC) No. 1331/2008 [on the common authorization procedure for food additives, food enzymes and food flavourings], Regulation (EC) No. 1107/2009 [on plant protection products] and Regulation (EU) No. 2015/2283 [on novel foods]. Available at: https://corporateeurope.org/sites/default/files/2019-04/Final%20compromise%20 text.pdf.

47 Grant W (2012). Agricultural Policy, Food Policy, and Communicable Disease Policy. *Journal of Health Politics, Policy and Law*, 37(6):1031–48.

Box 3.1 *International dimensions of food safety policy*

Sanitary and phytosanitary standards cover definitions and safe practices and are crucial to the operation of trade in food, plants, and animals. The European Union is embedded in the complex network of agreements that regulates these issues. That includes the Codex Alimentarius Commission, of which it and the member states are members and which sets basic food standards; the World Organisation for Animal Health (OIE), in which the Commission is a formal observer and the EU coordinates member state positions; and the International Plant Protection Convention, which all member states have signed and which focuses on pest control. It also includes extensive and detailed bilateral agreements. Trade agreements can affect all of these areas of regulation, e.g. permissible levels and kinds of pesticides or GMOs, which can make these seemingly technical issues very contentious (see 4.7 and Box 3.2 Food standards and trade agreements). The European Union is one of the key actors in these fields, influencing standards and procedures far beyond its borders.

---

agrifood industry). Implementing it is not just a technical challenge, though; the establishment of the system also meant "Europeanizing" very different and often well-established organizations and regulatory regimes.

The resulting system is complex and evolving.[48] Member States are responsible for policing each stage of the farm-to-fork chain according to legislated EU standards, as well as coordinating to cope with the problem of cross-border food movements (e.g. through implementing a livestock tracking scheme).

Policing cross-border food movement is both a *raison d'être* of EU food safety policy, since the added value of EU action is obvious and considerable, and a major challenge. In 2013's "Horsegate" scandal, for example, it emerged that horsemeat from Romania was being sold as beef by major supermarkets in the UK and Ireland. Further investigation found that the product had moved around five EU countries (Romania, France, Belgium, the UK, Ireland), partially orchestrated by a firm based in a sixth, the Netherlands, with investigators considering at least three Member States as the source of the meat as they tried to identify the stage at which it had been wrongly labelled, and by whom.[49] As a team of researchers concluded in 2017, "Horsegate raised the profile of food fraud and crime in supply chains and despite improvements to date, further

---

48 Caldeira S et al. (2016). Overview of the food chain system and the European regulatory framework in the fields of food safety and nutrition. European Commission. Available at: https://publications.europa.eu/en/publication-detail/-/publication/90b67c7b-9a92-11e6-9bca-01aa75ed71a1/language-en/format-PDF/source-search.

49 https://www.theguardian.com/uk/2013/feb/15/horsemeat-scandal-the-essential-guide. Eventually, the case led to the prosecution in Dutch courts of a Netherlands-based meat dealer whose warehouse was located in Belgium.

Box 3.2   *Food standards and trade agreements*

Why are Europeans concerned about chlorinated chicken and hormone-treated beef? The conclusion of the EU–Canada Comprehensive Economic Trade Agreement (CETA) and negotiations with the US on a possible Transatlantic Trade and Investment Agreement have been met with widespread protests that, among other objections, raise concerns about food safety standards in countries outside the EU and the potential for trade agreements to lower the quality of food available in the single market.

Chlorinated chicken and hormone-treated beef are not allowed to be sold within the EU. To date, the EU has supported trade policies which are in line with its internal commitment to supporting a high level of human, animal and plant life and health. But a high level of health in law does not guarantee a high level of health in practice.

Trading with countries that have different food safety standards presents several distinct challenges to balancing economic growth and health. First, officials have to formally agree on how their food standards will be treated in each other's legal jurisdictions. This negotiation process is highly detailed, politically sensitive and often not publicly accessible. The extent to which health is prioritized in negotiations depends on a combination of legal constraints and political pressures on the negotiators and their relative bargaining power. A lack of transparent information about proceedings can fuel concern among the public and public health advocates.

Once an agreement is in place, other countries (and, in the case of investment agreements, companies) can challenge its content through a number of dispute settlement mechanisms. Disputes can be lengthy and expensive and are not particularly transparent. The EU's positions on hormone-treated beef and chlorinated chicken have been the subjects of trade disputes within the WTO system, putting EU officials under pressure to change these policies. EU officials have, to date, resisted these pressures.

Furthermore, realizing food safety standards in practice rests upon national competences and capacities, with Member States responsible for conducting compliance checks on imported goods. Regardless of what is decided in a trade agreement, the reality of enforcement and compliance may not match up with the legal intent.

---

collaboration between industry and government is required in order to align fully with the recommendations."[50]

The governance structure that is set up to deal with this wide variety of issues is built at the Member State level through Member State implementation and enforcement of EU law, and coordination through EU-level mechanisms to manage cross-border movements. EFSA, the agency, is designed to be a source

---

50   Brooks S et al. (2017). Four years post-Horsegate: an update of measures and actions put in place following the horsemeat incident of 2013. *NPJ Science of Food*, 1(1):5.

of scientific advice and communication, rather than an executive agency making or implementing policy. This makes it closer to the ECDC, reliant on scientific expertise and credibility, than to EMA, which is a *de facto* regulator.[51] The Member States are the regulators and enforcers in this highly Europeanized area of policy.

3.1.5   Vaccination

Vaccination is one of the most cost-effective public health measures. Vaccines have contributed significantly to the control of communicable diseases worldwide, preventing 2.7 million people from contracting measles, 2 million from contracting neonatal tetanus and 1 million people from contracting pertussis each year. In Europe seasonal flu vaccinations prevent around 2 million people per year from contracting influenza. Vaccines are responsible for the eradication of smallpox and Europe's polio-free status.[52]

In recent years, however, the EU has experienced a number of serious outbreaks of vaccine-preventable diseases that are attributable to lower levels of vaccination coverage in the population. These outbreaks come with real health consequences, including the potential for severe complications that can lead to hospitalization or death.

Vaccination is certainly a public health issue of the first order across Europe, even if the real and potential EU role is not always appreciated. In terms of routine vaccination, coverage rates for certain vaccinations (e.g. against measles) have fallen below the level required to maintain herd immunity in some EU Member States. The reasons for the fall in coverage include failure to reach vulnerable groups of people within the population, increased vaccine hesitancy (a "delay in acceptance or refusal of vaccines despite availability of vaccine services") and deficiencies in organization, financing and provision within Member States' health systems.[53] Subpar herd immunity is thus a symptom of larger political and social problems, including income inequality and social exclusion, poor access to healthcare, low trust in governments and/or scientific evidence, and inadequately resourced or managed health services. There is, therefore, considerable variation in vaccination rates across the EU.

In particular, concerns have been raised in recent years about falling confidence in vaccination among members of the public and health professionals. The

---

51   Krapohl S (2004). Credible commitment in non-independent regulatory agencies: a comparative analysis of the European agencies for pharmaceuticals and foodstuffs. *European Law Journal*, 10(5):518–38.

52   European Commission (2018). Questions and Answers: EU Cooperation on Communicable Diseases. Available at: http://europa.eu/rapid/press-release_MEMO-18-3458_en.htm.

53   Rechel B, Richardson E, McKee M (2018). *The Organization and Delivery of Vaccine Services in the EU.* Copenhagen: WHO Regional office for Europe, on behalf of the European Observatory on Health Systems and Policies.

reasons for this decline in confidence are complex, with the fears and concerns of individuals being stoked by the spread of misinformation by the media and through social media channels, as well as by claims made by populist politicians in a variety of countries. In many cases, attitudes towards vaccination are influenced by the relationships of individuals and communities to governments, including both a lack of trust in policy-makers setting vaccine policy as well as distrust of government agents administering vaccinations at ground level. Pro-vaccination public health messages are often ineffective in the context of the strong emotional responses elicited by this combination of factors.[54] A further complication is an increase in hesitancy to promote vaccines among health professionals, which points to a gap between stated national policies and the attitudes of health professionals responsible for implementing these policies, e.g. pharmacists, nurses and doctors.[55]

The regulation of vaccines as products for sale in the single market is the responsibility of both the EU and Member States. This means that the approval of vaccines, along with pharmacovigilance (the act of monitoring the effects of a medical product after it enters the market and the reporting of adverse effects), fall under areas of shared competency.[56] Influenza vaccines for use in the single market must be authorized through a central procedure governed by the European Medicines Agency. In addition, most vaccine manufacturers choose to use this central route to obtain authorization for their other vaccines. Member States can also authorize vaccines, in which case the rules of mutual recognition apply, with a product authorized in one Member State automatically authorized for use across the single market. In the case of vaccination as a response to disease outbreaks, an emergency procedure is employed that allows vaccines to be pre-authorized in generic form and then more quickly authorized once a pandemic occurs (*see also* section 4.1.1 for an explanation of pharmacovigilance procedure).[57]

The procurement and use of vaccines are Member State competencies. In terms of policies governing vaccine use, there is significant variation by country. In response to measles, for example, vaccination is mandatory in nine Member States and voluntary in the other 19 countries. Other measures such as vaccine requirements for children entering the school system complicate this picture.[58] Vaccination policies also vary considerably by disease. In the case of adult influenza

---

54 Larson J et al. (2018). The State of Vaccine Confidence in the EU, *The Lancet*, 392(10161):2244–6.

55 Ibid.

56 De Ruijter A (2019). *EU Health Law and Policy: the Expansion of EU Power in Public Health and Health Care*. Oxford: Oxford University Press.

57 Hervey T, McHale J (2015). *European Union Health Law: Themes and Implications*. Cambridge: Cambridge University Press.

58 Rechel B, Richardson E, McKee M (2018). *The Organization and Delivery of Vaccine Services in the EU*. Copenhagen: WHO Regional office for Europe, on behalf of the European Observatory on Health Systems and Policies.

vaccinations, the EU has a generally subpar coverage rate, even among older, vulnerable populations, with some national variation.[59]

For these reasons, the EU institutions play a vital role in promoting recommended vaccinations in order to protect public health. In response to concerns about low coverage rates and decreased vaccine confidence, the Council recommended a series of EU actions to strengthen cooperation among Member States.[60] These actions include the collation and dissemination of data on vaccination rates and levels of confidence across the EU, evaluation of the feasibility of creating an EU-wide vaccination card, monitoring national policies and the creation of guidance that can inform them, technological solutions that enable interoperable data exchange of national vaccination records, the promotion of vaccination through a public awareness campaign, convening key pro-vaccination stakeholders, and measures to facilitate the joint procurement of vaccines, e.g. by exploring stockpiling and engaging collectively with vaccine manufacturers.

It remains to be seen to what extent these policies will be effective in addressing the concerns of public health officials with regard to falling coverage. The Commission has developed an action plan to implement the Council recommendations by 2022.[61] However, to the extent that anti-vaccination remains a politically popular position in Europe, we can expect some Member States to be themselves hesitant to act.

3.1.6   Joint procurement

Within the context of EU action to cross-border health threats (*see* section 3.1.3) a new tool was introduced to strengthen preparedness. With Decision No. 1082/2013/EU the possibility was introduced for Member States to engage on a voluntary basis in a procedure to jointly procure medical countermeasures, particularly vaccines (Article 5). This process was accelerated by the H1N1 flu pandemic in 2009, when countries were competing to purchase and stockpile available flu vaccine supplies and antiviral medication, for which they paid relatively high amounts without using them.[62] Both the Council and the European Parliament concluded that a joint procurement mechanism would help to improve

---

59   Ibid.

60   Council Recommendation of 7 December 2018 (2018/C 466/01) on strengthened cooperation against vaccine-preventable diseases.

61   European Commission (2019). "Roadmap for the implementation of actions by the European Commission based on the Commission Communication and the Council Recommendation on strengthening cooperation against vaccine preventable diseases". Available at: https://ec.europa.eu/health/sites/health/files/vaccination/docs/2019-2022_roadmap_en.pdf.

62   Nicoll A, McKee M (2010). Moderate pandemic, not many dead: learning the right lessons in Europe from the 2009 pandemic. *European Journal of Public Health*, 20(5):486–8.

the purchasing power of Member States and strengthen solidarity between them by ensuring equitable access.[63]

In 2014 the EU Joint Procurement Agreement (JAPE) was adopted and entered into force after 14 Member States had signed it. In June 2019 Bulgaria became the 25th Member State to join the agreement. The European Commission acts as the Permanent Secretariat, which is also in charge of the preparation and organization of the joint procurement procedure. For each procurement procedure, the technical specifications and allocation criteria are determined by a separate committee.[64]

The first joint procurement procedure was successfully concluded in 2016 for the Botulinum anti-toxin. In March 2019 framework contracts were signed between the 15 Member States, the Commission and a pharmaceutical company for the production and supply of pandemic influenza vaccines.[65] Procedures for other countermeasures, including personal protective equipment, are still under way. While the Decision leaves some discretion to Member States to determine the scope for joint procurement under the JAPE, it is by nature confined to medical countermeasures to address serious cross-border threats to health. This includes medicines, medical devices, services and goods that could be used to mitigate or treat a life-threatening or otherwise serious hazard to health from a biological, chemical, environmental or unknown origin which spreads, or entails a significant risk of spreading, across the national borders of Member States, and which may necessitate coordination at Union level in order to ensure a high level of human health protection.[66] These could include communicable diseases, bio toxins, chemical and environmental events.

Even if the current framework leaves negligible room for extending joint procurement beyond this scope, the idea of using it for other purposes has gained interest in recent years, especially in the context of the growing problem of high-priced medicines, which was triggered in 2014 with the Hepatitis C drug sofosbuvir. In a resolution adopted in 2017 the European Parliament called upon the Commission and the Council to develop new measures and tools that could help to ensure affordable patient access to medicines without having an

---

63 Council conclusions on Lessons learned from the A/H1N1 pandemic – Health security in the European Union, Brussels, 13 September 2010; European Parliament resolution of 8 March 2011 on Evaluation of the management of H1N1 influenza in 2009–2010 in the EU (2010/2153(INI)).

64 Azzopardi-Muscat N, Schroder-Back P, Brand H (2016). The European Union Joint Procurement Agreement for cross-border health threats: What is the potential for this new mechanism of health system collaboration? *Health Economics, Policy and Law*, 12(1):43–59.

65 European Commission (2019). Memo. Framework contracts for pandemic influenza vaccines 28 March 2019. Available at: https://ec.europa.eu/health/sites/health/files/preparedness_response/docs/ev_20190328_memo_en.pdf.

66 European Commission (2014). Medical countermeasures that could be procured in common under the Joint Procurement Agreement. December 2014.

unacceptable impact on public healthcare budgets, including voluntary joint procurements and voluntary cooperation in price negotiations. This avenue was further explored under the Maltese EU presidency in 2017, which drew attention to the specific challenges in purchasing health technologies for smaller populations and promoted the idea of enhanced voluntary cooperation between countries.[67] Various European countries have meanwhile engaged in regional collaborations, such as the BeNeLuxA initiative[68] (started in 2015) or the Valletta Declaration[69] (2017). These projects essentially aim at improving transparency, sharing experience and enhancing bargaining power for procurement agencies. They are focused on collaboration along the whole procurement process, from horizon scanning, through health technology assessment, to price negotiations.

3.1.7   Communicable diseases and threats to health

One of the most consistent areas of EU health action has been on communicable disease and other cross-border threats to health.[70] The logic is inexorable. Spillover from an increasingly integrated Europe creates incentives to coordinate knowledge and responses; integration means population movements and supply chains and, as a result, infectious diseases can cross borders. Coordination and integration in the area of communicable disease control is nonetheless very difficult. The starting points in different Member States are very varied, with different organizations, resources and skills.[71]

Politically, communicable disease control policy is caught in the logic of crisis and collective action: outside of crises, it is hard to find energy for collective action, whereas in crises, countries can sometimes overcome the barriers to collective measures and take actions (in others, they merely fall into recriminations and local initiatives).

---

67   Espin J et al. (2017). How can voluntary cross-border collaboration in public procurement improve access to health technologies in Europe? Policy Brief 21, Copenhagen: WHO Regional office for Europe, on behalf of the European Observatory on Health Systems and Policies.

68   http://www.beneluxa.org/collaboration.

69   https://www.southeusummit.com/about/valletta-declaration/.

70   See the 2012 special issue on the subject: *Journal of Health Politics, Policy and Law*, 37(6); de Ruijter A. *EU Health Law & Policy: The Expansion of EU Power in Public Health and Health Care*. Oxford University Press, 2019.

71   Elliott H, Jones DK, Greer SL (2012). Mapping infectious disease control in the European Union. *Journal of Health Politics, Policy and Law*, 37(6):935–54; Reintjes R (2012). Variation matters: epidemiological surveillance in Europe. *Journal of Health Politics, Policy and Law*, 37(6):955–65; Reintjes R et al. (2007). Benchmarking national surveillance systems: a new tool for the comparison of communicable disease surveillance and control in Europe. *European Journal of Public Health*, 17(4):375–80; Greer SL, Mätzke M (2012). Bacteria without borders: communicable disease politics in Europe. *Journal of Health Politics, Policy and Law*, 37(6):815–914. We would like to thank Anniek de Ruijter for her comments on this section.

Protection against health threats, accordingly, creates a combination of pressure for and constraint on European integration. On the one hand, the subject matter of diseases and health threats including bioterrorism is an inherent cross-border issue where the EU has complementary legislative competence to coordinate Member States' responses.[72] Both infectious disease outbreaks (including SARS and influenza in recent years) affect multiple European countries. This is a case for coordination, particularly given that Member States' capacity for risk assessment and management is variable. On the other hand, Member States have very different infrastructures, resources and politics and are not always willing to cooperate, particularly as they retain competence with respect to national healthcare budgets.[73] The result is that the EU has taken some decisive steps into control of communicable diseases, but it has not been granted the full range of powers that are associated with a coherent communicable disease control and response system.

Monitoring and surveillance of communicable diseases

Beginning in the 1980s the EU began to fund research, training and disease-specific monitoring networks, and this evolved into a network for monitoring and surveillance of communicable diseases, formalized in 1998.[74] However, this overarching network had evolved from a series of disease-specific networks and depended on ad hoc coordination between national authorities, coordinated by the Commission. The anthrax alerts of 2001 in the United States combined with the sudden global spread of the virus causing SARS in 2003, followed by pandemic influenza threats, abruptly focused attention on the weaknesses of these arrangements, and a specialist agency, the ECDC, was established instead to coordinate surveillance and monitoring of communicable disease.[75]

Reflecting the wider distribution of health powers between the EU and Member States, the ECDC has not become a single European centre in the same way as the Centers for Disease Control and Prevention (CDC) have in the United States. Rather, Europe has adopted the already existing network approach that was developed under Commission auspices, with the ECDC acting as a focal point of

---

72   TFEU, Article 168(1).
73   TFEU, Article 168(7).
74   European Parliament and Council (1998). Decision No. 2119/98/EC setting up a network for the epidemiological surveillance and control of communicable diseases in the Community, *Official Journal*, L 268/1; Greer SL (2017). "Constituting Public Health Surveillance in Twenty-First Century Europe", in Weimer M & de Ruijter A (eds). *Regulating Risks in the European Union: The Co-Production of Expert and Executive Power*. London: Bloomsbury; de Ruijter A (2013). *Uncovering European Health Law*. Amsterdam: University of Amsterdam.
75   European Parliament and Council (2004). Regulation (EC) No. 851/2004 establishing a European centre for disease prevention and control. *Official Journal*, L 142/1; Greer SL (2012). The European Centre for Disease Prevention and Control: hub or hollow core? *Journal of Health Politics, Policy and Law*, 37(6):1001–30.

surveillance undertaken by the Member States. While this means that the number of staff of the ECDC (around 300) is small in comparison with the American CDC, it is an order of magnitude larger than the couple of dozen staff formerly responsible for communicable diseases in the European Commission, and indeed more than the entire public health directorate of the European Commission. It is not directly charged with risk management, which remains overwhelmingly the job of Member States. Its job is surveillance and risk assessment, plus to some extent developing public communication strategies. However, in recent years, in the context of particular regional crises, the ECDC has also developed some operational capabilities and from time to time sends its public health specialists to affected areas to report directly on the ground. Developing a role in the crowded and very political world of European communicable disease control is a challenge, and EU-level action can be overshadowed by failures in Member States' risk management and response systems. Like so much of European policy, the ECDC relies on networks of scientists as well as international organizations, and its effectiveness rests in its own effectiveness at inspiring and using them.

Managing and responding to threats

The responsibilities of the ECDC are centred in monitoring and surveillance, and to some extent capacity building and research. The responsibility for the policy response to threats to health has primarily been kept by the Member States and the core EU institutions and is, in the first instance, the responsibility of a "Health Security Committee",[76] which addresses issues such as preparedness and response for public health emergencies, as well as coordinating responses in crisis situations. The Health Security Committee's evolution has been interesting; many of its functions today accumulated informally as Member State officials found it was a useful venue to coordinate their activities.

Historically, crisis response and management has been the weak point of European action on health threats. Faced with urgent situations and domestic pressures, Member State governments have tended to revert to taking national measures, sometimes even against the interests of other Member States. The ECDC's visibility is not matched with legal powers or capabilities to intervene, and even the Commission has limited ability to coordinate what Member States do. This was demonstrated all too clearly during the swine flu pandemic in 2009, when several Member States bought what influenza vaccine and antiviral medications

---

76 European Parliament and Council (2013). Decision No. 1082/2013/EU on serious cross-border threats to health and repealing Decision 2119/98/EC. Luxembourg: Publications Office of the European Union; de Ruijter A (2013). *Uncovering European health law* [thesis]. Faculty of Law, University of Amsterdam.

they could, and declined to share. This episode gave rise to joint procurement as an EU policy instrument.[77]

3.1.8   Civil protection: RescEU and the European Medical Corps

Global and European health challenges increasingly include health or other emergencies such as new disease outbreaks, large forest fires and other natural disasters associated with human-induced climate change, as well as longstanding threats such as a radiological accident.[78] The increased tempo – and increased likelihood – of such disasters is the justification for the EU's increasingly developed civil protection mechanisms.

The Civil Protection Mechanism, operative since 2001, is a mechanism for the coordination and strengthening of Member States' relief capacities in action as well as in disaster preparedness and training. Initially primarily used for disaster relief outside the EU, it has increasingly operated inside the EU for civil protection crises beyond the capabilities of individual Member States. It has been activated to respond to the refugees arriving in 2015, Mediterranean forest fires in 2017 and forest fires in Sweden in 2018. Its future planning indicates that it will continue to have a role within the EU, notably with investment in firefighting equipment and expertise. It has marshalled and shared resources from firefighting equipment to sophisticated satellite geospatial data (through the Copernicus Emergency Management Service) to search and rescue teams in its eighteen years of existence.

In March 2019 the mechanism was upgraded and renamed RescEU.[79] It is based on Article 196 TFEU, which mandates that the EU shall help coordinate Member State civil protection, and Article 214 TFEU, which authorizes the EU to assist victims of natural or human-caused disasters worldwide. The Civil Protection Pool is the register of assets that Member States[80] make available to RescEU activities. These specialized assets are certified as suitable and engage in regular exercises in order to ensure that they can be deployed and work together. They are only deployed on EU activities by their Member States after a request from the Civil Protection Mechanism. The Emergency Response Coordination Centre acts as a hub for requests and coordination. In other words, it remains under

---

77   European Commission (2019). Memo. Framework contracts for pandemic influenza vaccines 28 March 2019. Available at: https://ec.europa.eu/health/sites/health/files/preparedness_response/docs/ev_20190328_memo_en.pdf.

78   The EURATOM Treaty to this day is separate from the other EU treaties and there is no interest in integrating it. This means that the legal structure for handling radiological threats to health is different, but in practice the formal and informal weight of the EU mechanisms means that EU preparation and practice guide planning for radiological as well as other threats.

79   Decision (EU) 2019/420 of the European Parliament and of the Council of 13 March 2019 amending Decision No. 1313/2013/EU on a European Union Civil Protection Mechanism.

80   And Iceland, Norway, Serbia, North Macedonia, Montenegro and Turkey.

Member State control, but with a slowly increasing degree of Europeanization coming through coordination, joint planning, joint preparation and exercises, and joint service in crises.

The Civil Protection Pool includes the European Medical Corps, which was set up in the aftermath of the 2014 Ebola outbreak in West Africa and began operating in February 2016.[81] It is the EU's principal contribution to the WHO's Global Health Emergency Workforce initiative, which seeks to certify the competency and identify the types of medical resources needed in an emergency and thereby improve matching (ensuring that the right expertise and equipment arrives) and ensure quality among the diverse groups, including civil society and governments, that might have willingness to help and useful resources. The EMC initiative is closely coordinated with the WHO initiative.

RescEU and civil protection in general will be an issue to watch. On one hand, Member States jealously guard their autonomy and resources, in principle and in practice. On the other hand, in the face of natural and human-caused disasters in an increasingly integrated EU, and an increasingly threatening global climate, there is a case for coordination, joint work and even pooled resources. The creation of the civil protection machinery reflects the case for joint working even if its effectiveness and evolution remain to be established.

3.1.9   Substances of human origin

Many changes in public health systems and policies come about not through carefully considered development but rather in response to specific crises, as has already been discussed with communicable diseases. One specifically European aspect to this is that sometimes national governments see an advantage in passing responsibility for problematic issues to the European level; as well as pooling policy and technical resources, there is safety in numbers through acting at European level – whatever decisions are made, at least everyone is in it together. Substances of human origin is such an example. The original health article introduced in the Maastricht Treaty in 1992 did not include powers for European legislation on this topic; the choice by Member States to add such powers through the Amsterdam Treaty in 1997 reflected national problems, in particular the HIV-contaminated blood scandal in France in the 1980s, as well as perceived gaps in the regulatory regime for substances of human origin in comparison, for example, with the developing regulations for medicinal products.[82]

---

81 Pariat M (2016). Europe's medical emergency response. *Crisis Response Journal*, 11:3. Available at: https://ec.europa.eu/echo/sites/echo-site/files/europes_medical_emergency_response.pdf.

82 Tabuteau D (2007). La sécurité sanitaire, réforme institutionnelle ou résurgence des politiques de santé publique? *Les Tribunes de la santé*, 16(3):87–103.

The development of legislation on blood also illustrated another dynamic of EU policy development: the way in which discussions in other forums are used to develop and build consensus first, and only afterwards is actual legislation brought forward, coming at the end of a much longer process. In this case, the Council of Europe acted as an antechamber for the legislation ultimately proposed by the Commission, drawing on a long history of developing European standards in this area.[83]

The actual legislation on blood, blood products, tissues and cells itself is relatively limited, reflecting the narrow treaty mandate.[84] It is focused on setting minimum standards for quality and safety, such as oversight of providers, traceability and notification of adverse incidents, and a range of technical requirements. The legislation notably does not set requirements to ensure self-sufficiency in blood for the EU, despite this being part of the original set of objectives identified by the Member States;[85] this reflects the perennial concern of national administrations about granting powers to the EU relating to the organization of their health systems.[86] The European Commission carried out in 2017 and 2018 the first formal evaluation of the EU blood, tissues and cells legislation since the adoption of the basic Acts in 2002 (on blood), and 2004 (tissues and cells).[87]

The background to European action on organs, however, is a more positive one; a shiningly good example in one country (Spain) regarding organ transplantation providing the inspiration for collective action at European level to try to overcome the persistent shortage in organs for transplantation that affects Europe.[88] Accordingly, the EU action in this area is much broader than the specific legislation on quality and safety; it also encompasses a wider action

---

83 Faber J-C (2004). The European Blood Directive: a new era of blood regulation has begun. *Transfusion Medicine*, 14(4):257–73; Farrell A-M (2005). "The emergence of EU governance in public health: the case of blood policy and regulation", in Steffen M (ed.). *Health governance in Europe: issues, challenges and theories*. Abingdon: Routledge, pp.134–51; Steffen M (2012). The Europeanization of public health: how does it work? The seminal role of the AIDS case. *Journal of Health Politics, Policy and Law*, 37(6):1057–89.

84 Article 168 (4): "The European Parliament and the Council … shall … adopt: (a) measures setting high standards of quality and safety of organs, and substances of human origin, blood and blood derivatives; these measures shall not prevent any Member States from maintaining or introducing more stringent protective measures."

85 Council of the European Union (1996). *Council resolution of 12 November 1996 on a strategy towards blood safety and self-sufficiency in the European Community (96/C 374/01)*. Luxembourg: Publications Office of the European Communities.

86 Article. 168 (7): "These measures (para 4(a)) shall not affect national provisions on the donation or medical use of organs and blood."

87 European Commission. Evaluation of the EU blood, tissues and cells legislation. Available at: https://ec.europa.eu/health/blood_tissues_organs/policy/evaluation_en.

88 DG for Health and Consumers (2008). *Staff Working Document SEC(2008)2956: impact assessment and annexes accompanying the proposal for a directive on quality and safety of organ donation and transplantation and action plan*. Luxembourg: Publications Office of the European Communities; Greer SL (2016). "Intergovernmental governance for health: federalism, decentralization and communicable diseases", in Greer SL, Wismar M & Figueras J (eds.). *Strengthening Health System Governance: Better Policies, Stronger Performance*. McGraw Hill Education and Open University Press, Berkshire, pp. 187–205.

plan aimed at increasing organ availability and enhancing the efficiency and accessibility of transplantation systems, as well as supporting improvements in quality and safety.[89]

3.1.10 Health in all policies

There is extensive evidence about the importance of factors beyond health for health itself and, therefore, there is a need for health issues to be taken into account in other areas of public policy.[90] This has been a part of the European approach to health since the introduction of the specific article on health into the treaties, with its requirement (strengthened over the years) that health protection requirements be integrated throughout the EU's action. The EU has a history of adopting principles that are to be taken into account across government, such as the precautionary principle, health in all policies, or less obviously useful ones such as the "innovation principle", which was backed by a coalition of chemicals, tobacco and other industries which have an interest in allowing greater risks from their products, to public health and in general.[91]

Alongside the Commission's initial strategy for implementing its new treaty mandate on health in 1993, the Commission took internal steps to ensure the integration of health into other policies:[92]

- the reinforcement of interservice consultation prior to Commission decisions whenever a decision might have implications for public health;

- the setting up of an Inter-Service Group on Health to ensure mutual exchange of information and internal coordination with regard to health and health protection aspects of policies and legislative proposals

as well as publishing annual reports on this process of integration. However, although initially voluminous and covering a wide range of potential impacts,

---

89 European Commission (2008). *Communication on an action plan on organ donation and transplantation (2009–2015): strengthened cooperation between Member States (COM(2008)819)*. Luxembourg: Publications Office of the European Communities.

90 Ståhl T et al. (eds.) (2006). *Health in all policies: prospects and potentials*. Helsinki: Ministry of Social Affairs and Health.

91 The European Parliament passed this in 2019. Its principal backers were in the European Risk Forum, which hides its membership and purports to be a think tank focused on excellence in risk management. The innovation principle is that any regulation should consider its impact on "innovation" as a competitor to, for example, the precautionary principle (Box 3.3): https://esharp.eu/debates/innovation/the-innovation-principle. This will present another hurdle to, for example, regulation of innovative tobacco products such as heat-not-burn, or to regulation of novel chemicals in the food system. As with Health in All Policies, though, its actual impact will depend on how seriously the Commission takes it, and how much pressure the Council and Parliament put on it to take it seriously.

92 European Commission (1995). *Report on the integration of health protection requirements in Community policies (COM(95)196)*. Brussels: European Commission, p. iii.

the reports became shorter and less regular,[93] and ultimately the Commission decided to abandon providing regular reports on the overall integration of health protection requirements across European policies in 1999. Instead, attention turned to developing methodologies for assessing the impact of the EU on health, with the Commission funding development of a methodology that could be used for health impact assessment at European level,[94] as well as a specific impact assessment tool for impact on health systems.[95]

However, by then the overall approach within the Commission had changed. Health was not the only area that the treaties required to be taken into account across other policies; other objectives such as the environment, consumer protection, culture, regional policy, animal welfare and development cooperation also had their own "integration clauses", which led to a proliferation of impact assessments and methodologies. There was also increasing pressure on the Commission to consider all the impacts of its proposals more carefully and to do so in a systematic way. The Commission responded by replacing these different sector-specific impact assessments with a single integrated impact assessment process covering all the different dimensions of a proposal's potential impact, grouped under the three headings of economic, social and environmental impact;[96] impacts on health were included under the "social" pillar, and the tools developed specifically for assessing impact on health and health systems became just a part of this wider evaluation.

The process for evaluating these impact assessments was then further strengthened in 2006 with the establishment of an internal Impact Assessment Board within the Commission,[97] which would review impact assessments of proposals before they were submitted to the Commission for adoption. This Board is made up of senior officials from the central Secretariat-General and the DGs with relevant economic, environmental and social expertise; there is no member from DG SANTE. However, despite this strengthening of the process, an evaluation for

---

93 *See* the *Integration of health protection requirements in Community policies.* Second Report (COM(96)407) of 1996, Third Report (COM(1998)34) of 1998 and Fourth Report (not officially issued by the Commission, but produced in 1999; available at: http://ec.europa.eu/health/ph_overview/Documents/ke03_en.pdf, accessed 4 July 2014.

94 European Commission (2001). *European policy health impact assessment.* Available at: http://ec.europa.eu/health/ph_projects/2001/monitoring/monitoring_project_2001_full_en.htm#11, accessed 4 July 2014; *European policy health impact assessment guide.* Available at: http://ec.europa.eu/health/ph_projects/2001/monitoring/fp_monitoring_2001_a6_frep_11_en.pdf, accessed 4 July 2014. Brussels: European Commission.

95 European Commission (2004). *Policy health impact assessment for the European Union.* Brussels: European Commission. Available at: http://ec.europa.eu/health/ph_projects/2001/monitoring/monitoring_project_2001_full_en.htm#11, accessed 28 July 2014.

96 European Commission (2002). *Communication on impact assessment (COM(2002)276).* Brussels: European Commission, 2002.

97 European Commission (2014). *Impact Assessment Board.* Brussels: European Commission. Available at: http://ec.europa.eu/smart-regulation/impact/iab/iab_en.htm, accessed 4 July 2014.

Box 3.3   *The precautionary principle*

The precautionary principle in EU law is in Article 191, the article on environmental protection, but its scope covers all EU policy including consumer protection, health and animal and plant health. The principle is well known in environmental and regulatory policy debates. Crudely, it focuses on identifying risks *ex-ante* (before something is released onto the market) and is often counterposed to a view associated with the US that emphasizes *ex-post* demonstrated risks.

The Commission defined its scope and procedures for application in a 2000 Communication.[a] Its scope is: "where preliminary objective scientific evaluation indicates that there are reasonable grounds for concern that the potentially dangerous effects on the environment, human, animal or plant health may be inconsistent with the high level of protection chosen for the Community". The procedures that it then requires, according to the Communication, are "measures based on the precautionary principle", which should be, inter alia:

- proportional to the chosen level of protection,
- non-discriminatory in their application,
- consistent with similar measures already taken,
- based on an examination of the potential benefits and costs of action or lack of action (including, where appropriate and feasible, an economic cost/benefit analysis),
- subject to review, in the light of new scientific data, and
- capable of assigning responsibility for producing the scientific evidence necessary for a more comprehensive risk assessment.

As might be expected, in the subsequent eighteen years arguments about the precautionary principle, its implementation by the EU, Member States and courts, and the specifics of different policy areas have flourished. Nonetheless, it is a meaningfully different starting point from the US or Chinese approach and it gives the EU a different underlying set of legal constraints in developing policies in areas with unknown health risks. Much of the criticism of the EU approach, like criticism of the often different US approach, should actually be aimed at the slowness of its legislative procedures, legalism and consequent rigidity in the face of quickly changing technologies such as synthetic biology.[b]

[a]   Communication from the Commission on the precautionary principle /* COM/2000/0001 final */

[b]   Greer SL, Trump B. Regulation and regime: the comparative politics of adaptive regulation in synthetic biology. Policy Sciences. Online Publication 2019. https://doi.org/10.1007/s11077-019-09356-0. For a broader perspective on EU risk regulation, *see* Weimer M, de Ruijter A (eds.). (2017) *Regulating risks in the European Union: The co-production of expert and executive power.* Oxford: Bloomsbury Publishing.

Box 3.4 *Antimicrobial resistance*

One area where the different powers of the European Union related to health can come together effectively is in tackling antimicrobial resistance. The Commission's "One Health Action Plan against Antimicrobial Resistance (AMR)"[a] sets out an integrated approach to tackling the issue for both human health and animal health, drawing on the EU's powers to address both and the links between use of antibiotics in animals and in humans. It outlines a range of actions involving better monitoring and surveillance, coordination across the EU and supporting prevention and control through more prudent use of antibiotics in both people and animals, as well as more research, and the EU is pushing for stronger global action. Nevertheless, high levels of certain types of AMR remain in the EU,[b] and the variations between countries in their rates suggest that there is still much work to be done in addressing the challenge within the EU.

[a] *See* https://ec.europa.eu/health/amr/sites/amr/files/amr_action_plan_2017_en.pdf.

[b] European Centre for Disease Prevention and Control (2018). Surveillance of antimicrobial resistance in Europe – Annual report of the European Antimicrobial Resistance Surveillance Network (EARS-Net) 2017. Stockholm: ECDC.

---

the Commission reported that the impact assessment process was not generally viewed internally as a credible or impartial one, being perceived by Commission officials more as an exercise in justifying the proposals concerned.[98] Externally, doubts have also been expressed about how far health impacts are really assessed in these integrated impact assessments.[99]

There is also a fundamental structural issue, which is the nature of European legislation. While regulations have direct effect, and their impact could in principle be assessed up front, the ultimate impact of directives depends substantially on how they are implemented by Member States into national legislation – a process that can vary quite substantially and puts in doubt how far it is actually possible for the European Commission to know the impact of proposals that have such national variability built in by design. Nevertheless, this process of understanding the impacts of other policies on health is a vital one, as the impact of other areas of European action on health is in many ways larger than the impact of the EU's actions that have health as a specific objective.

---

98 Evaluation Partnership (2007). *Evaluation of the Commission's impact assessment system: final report.* Executive Summary. Brussels: European Commission. Available at: http://ec.europa.eu/smart-regulation/impact/key_docs/docs/tep_eias_final_report_executive_summary_en.pdf, accessed 4 July 2014.

99 Koivusalo M (2010). The state of health in all policies (HiAP) in the European Union: potential and pitfalls. *Journal of Epidemiology and Community Health*, 64(6):500–3; Smith KE et al. (2010). Is the increasing policy use of impact assessment in Europe likely to undermine efforts to achieve healthy public policy? *Journal of Epidemiology and Community Health*, 64(6):478–87; Passarani I (2019). "Role of Evidence in the Formulation of European Public Health Policies". PhD thesis, Maastricht University.

3.2 Environment

As set by the treaties, the EU has broad objectives for the environment, which includes health:[100]

> European Union policy on the environment shall contribute to pursuit of the following objectives:
>
> preserving, protecting and improving the quality of the environment,
>
> *protecting human health,*
>
> prudent and rational utilization of natural resources, and
>
> promoting measures at international level to deal with regional or worldwide environmental problems, and in particular combating climate change [emphasis added].

The powers to achieve this objective are wide ranging (unlike the health article), although they require unanimity in the Council for some topics such as town and county planning and measures affecting the general structure of energy supply for a country.[101] Like health, environment also has an "integration clause", requiring environmental protection requirements to be integrated throughout the EU's policies and activities.[102]

Reflecting the broad powers in the treaties for environmental objectives, the EU has a formidable body of legislation and action on the environment, much of which also directly helps to improve human health. EU measures include legislation covering air and water quality, noise, chemicals and waste, as well as a wide range of other topics, with well over a hundred different directives, regulations and decisions.[103] The central importance of such environmental protection is illustrated by some of the links between health and environmental factors shown in Table 3.3; indeed, the World Health Organization estimates that environmental causes account for 18–20% of the overall burden of disease throughout the WHO European region – more in the eastern than in the western part covered by the EU.[104]

---

100 TFEU, Article 191, paragraph 1.
101 TFEU, Article 192.
102 TFEU, Article 11.
103 European Commission (2003). *Handbook on the implementation of EC environmental legislation.* Luxembourg: Publications Office of the European Union. Available at: http://ec.europa.eu/environment/enlarg/pdf/handbook_impl_ec_envi_legisl.pdf, accessed 4 July 2014.
104 European Environment Agency (2010). *The European environment: state and outlook 2010 – synthesis.* Luxembourg: Publications Office of the European Union.

Table 3.3 *Some health impacts and associations with environmental and lifestyle factors*

Health impact	Association with some environmental exposures
Infectious diseases	Water
	Air and food contamination
	Climate change-related changes in pathogen lifecycles
Cancer	Air pollution (PMs, mainly ≤PM2.5)
	Smoking and ETS
	Some pesticides
	Asbestos
	Natural toxins (aflatoxin)
	Polycyclic aromatic hydrocarbons (e.g. in diesel fumes)
	Some metals (e.g. arsenic, cadmium, chromium)
	Radiation (including sunlight)
	Radon
	Dioxins
Cardiovascular diseases	Air pollution (carbon monoxide, ground-level ozone, PMs)
	Smoking and ETS
	Lead
	Noise
	Inhalable particles
	Food (e.g. high cholesterol)
	Stress
Respiratory diseases including asthma	Smoking and ETS
	Air pollution (sulphur dioxide, nitrogen dioxide, ground-level ozone, $PM_{2.5}$ and PM_{10})
	Fungal spores
	Dust mites
	Pollen
	Pet hairs
	Skin and excreta
	Damp
Skin diseases	Ultraviolet radiation
	Some metals (e.g. nickel)
	Pentachlorophenol
	Dioxins
Diabetes, obesity	Foods (e.g. high fat)
	Poor exercise levels
Reproductive dysfunctions	PCBs
	DDT
	Cadmium
	Phthalates
	Endocrine disruptors
	Pharmaceuticals

Health impact	Association with some environmental exposures
Developmental (fetal and childhood) disorders	Metals (cadmium, lead, mercury)
	Smoking and ETS
	Some pesticides
	Endocrine disruptors
Nervous system disorders	Metals (lead, manganese)
	Methyl mercury
	Some solvents
	Organophosphates
Immune dysfunction	Ultraviolet-B radiation
	Some pesticides
Increased chemical sensitivity	Multiple chemical exposures at low doses

Source: EPHA (2008). Report on the status of health in the European Union: towards a healthier Europe (EUGLOREH Project).Brussels: DG Health and Consumers. Available at: http://ec.europa.eu/health/reports/publications/index_en.htm, accessed 28 July 2014; summary at http://www.epha.org/spip.php?article3439.

Notes: ETS: Environmental tobacco smoke; PCBs: Polychlorinated biphenyls; PM: Particulate matter.

Despite the progress made in many areas, challenges remain for environmental impact on health.[105] For example, for air pollutants there has been progress with some factors (such as sulphur dioxide and lead), but exposure to particulate matter and ground-level ozone is still causing significant ill-health. Another example concerns chemicals; although the EU's REACH legislation puts in place a detailed system of oversight for individual chemicals, there has been increasing concern about the real-world impact of cumulative exposure to many different chemicals over time.

3.2.1 Climate change

The specific issue of climate change is also relevant for health. Not only does climate change result in crop failures, which have an impact on nutrition, but many human diseases have been linked to climate fluctuations, including cardiovascular disease, respiratory illness in heatwaves and changes in the transmission of infectious, especially vector-borne, diseases such as malaria.[106] In 2009 the Commission published a working paper on the health impacts of

---

105 European Environment Agency (2010). *The European environment: state and outlook 2010 – synthesis*. Luxembourg: Publications Office of the European Union.

106 Patz JA, Thomson MC (2018) Climate change and health: Moving from theory to practice. *PLoS Med* 15(7): e1002628; Hotez PJ (2016) Neglected Tropical Diseases in the Anthropocene: The Cases of Zika, Ebola, and Other Infections. *PLoS Negl Trop Dis* 10(4): e0004648.

climate change,[107] which identified heat-related morbidity and mortality as the primary concern when assessing the impact of climate change on health; changes in the transmission of food- and vector-borne diseases will also emerge as health threats and will interact with other public health issues, such as migration, movement of staff and cross-border healthcare. This underlines the relevance of the EU's work on climate change more generally for health.

Given the importance of EU environmental protection for health, therefore, the relative lack of attention to this contribution to public health in Europe (e.g. in research) is surprising. This is perhaps because of the organizational factors discussed in chapter 2; the EU's environmental action is not led by the "health" part of the European Commission but rather by the "environment" department (and as of 2010 also a specific DG for action on climate change).[108] This organizational issue perhaps leads its vital contribution to improving human health to be overlooked by health stakeholders, both in terms of research and in terms of engagement by the wider health community.

3.2.2　An example: fine particle pollution

The scope and breadth of EU environmental policy is far beyond what we can discuss in this book. This section provides merely one timely example of EU environmental policy action with health benefits: fine particle pollution. Although air quality has improved in the EU over the last decades, the quality of life of many EU citizens remains hampered due to poor air quality, especially in urban areas.[109] The EU's action to improve air quality is based on three main pillars:[110] the ambient air quality standards set out in the Ambient Air Quality Directives (EU 2004, 2008) that require countries to adopt and implement air quality plans; the national emission reduction targets established in the National Emission Ceilings Directive (EU, 2016) that requires Member States to develop National Air Pollution Control Programmes by 2019 to comply with their emission reduction commitments; and emission standards that were set out in 2015 in EU legislation targeting industrial emissions, vehicles and transport fuels, etc.[111] In addition to these directives, the Clean Air Programme

---

107 European Commission (2009). *Staff Working Document: human, animal and plant health impacts of climate change (COM(2009) 147 final)*. Brussels: European Commission. Available at: http://ec.europa.eu/health/archive/ph_threats/climate/docs/com_2009-147_en.pdf, accessed 4 July 2014.

108 Although there is an integrated approach set out by the European Commission (2003). *European environment and health strategy (COM(2003)338)*. Brussels: European Commission. The treaty base for action on climate change is in large part the environmental treaty Article, 191.

109 European Commission (2018). Communication from the Commission to the European Parliament, the Council, the European Economic and Social Committee and the Committee of the Regions. 'A Europe that protects: Clean Air for all' (released 17 May 2018).

110 Ibid.

111 European Environment Agency(2018). Air quality in Europe – 2018 report. Luxembourg: Publications Office of the European Union, p. 15.

for Europe (CAPE), adopted in 2013, seeks to ensure full compliance with existing legislation by 2020. In 2018 the European Commission published its first clean air outlook in which it recognized action must be taken urgently in order to achieve the objectives set out in the Ambient Air Quality Directives at all governance levels.[112]

3.3   Health and safety at work

The large Title in the TFEU called "social policy" is substantially about what we might otherwise call labour law and equalities legislation. In terms of impact on health, it operates through several different mechanisms.

3.3.1   Occupational health and safety

Among the EU's list of social policy objectives, the first objective is "improvement in particular of the working environment to protect workers' health and safety".[113] The powers provided are broad in scope but quite specific in their nature, being limited to "directives, minimum requirements for gradual implementation, having regard to the conditions and technical rules obtaining in each of the Member States. Such directives shall avoid imposing administrative, financial and legal constraints in a way which would hold back the creation and development of small and medium-sized undertakings."[114]

The health and safety at work powers of the treaties described above have given rise to an extensive set of requirements to protect health at work. As well as the overall framework directive on safety and health at work, there is a wide range of detailed and sectoral provisions. Two European agencies – the European Agency for Safety and Health at Work and the European Foundation for Living and Working Conditions – also support the implementation of European action in this area. As described in section 3.3.3, this includes a directive on sharps (e.g. safe handling of needles and other products that can pose a hazard to workers)[115] specifically focused on workers in the health sector, although many of the other provisions are also highly relevant to healthcare workers.[116]

Finally, the Council formally adopted the Regulation establishing the European Labour Authority on June 13, 2019. This new Authority will ensure that Union

---

112 Ibid., p. 17.
113 TFEU, Article 153, paragraph 1(a).
114 TFEU, Article 153, paragraph 2(b).
115 Council of the European Union (2010). *Directive 2010/32/EU on prevention from sharp injuries in the hospital and healthcare sector of 10 May 2010 implementing the framework agreement on prevention from sharp injuries in the hospital and healthcare sector concluded by HOSPEEM and EPSU*. Luxembourg: Publications Office of the European Union.
116 European Commission (2011). *Occupational health and safety risks in the healthcare sector*. Luxembourg: Publications Office of the European Union.

rules on labour mobility are enforced in a fair, simple and effective way. More specifically, the Labour Authority will be responsible for supporting Member States in facilitating access to information for individuals and employers about their rights and obligations in the areas of labour mobility and social security coordination ; for supporting operational cooperation between national authorities in the cross-border enforcement of relevant Union law, including facilitating joint inspections; and for providing mediation and facilitate solutions in cases of disputes between national authorities.[117]

3.3.2   Working Time Directive

As part of the drive towards the integrated market launched by the Single European Act, there was concern that this should not be a "race to the bottom" for workers, with countries competing to become more competitive by lowering employment standards. Reflecting this, in 1990 the Commission proposed setting minimum standards for certain aspects of working time, in particular a minimum of 11 hours of rest per 24-hour period and specific protection for night workers and shift workers.[118] The directive was controversial, at least in the United Kingdom, which unsuccessfully tried to contest the original directive before the CJEU.[119] Health ministries also had mixed feelings about the proposal. On the one hand, protecting workers against long hours would help to ensure good health; on the other hand, health systems were themselves dependent on historical practices of long hours being worked by junior doctors. The directive as agreed in 1993 reflected this,[120] excluding doctors in training from these protections and allowing more general exceptions to be made for hospitals (as well as for some other sectors such as transport and sea fishing).

This exemption was intended to give time to find solutions to also protect these excluded categories of workers. The situation of doctors in training was given particular attention, with work for the Commission identifying a range of options that Member States could take,[121] including reorganizing work patterns, having some routine clinical work and administrative work undertaken by other staff such as senior nurses, improving retention of doctors in training who currently leave career grades, recruiting more junior doctors and sharing the workload

117 European Commission. "Statement. European Labour Authority ready to start working in October as decision is taken on new seat." Luxembourg, 13 June 2019

118 Commission of the European Communities (1990). *Proposal for a Council directive concerning certain aspects of the organization of working time (COM(90)317 final)*. Luxembourg: Publications Office of the European Union.

119 European Court of Justice. Case C-84/94 *United Kingdom v Council of the European Union*.

120 Council of the European Union (1993). Council Directive 93/104/EC concerning certain aspects of the organization of working time. *Official Journal*, L 307:18–24.

121 Cambridge Policy Consultants. *Business impact assessment – working time: excluded sectors: supplementary report: doctors in training*. Cambridge: Cambridge Policy Consultants. Available at: http://ec.europa.eu/social/BlobServlet?docid=2434&langid=en, accessed 4 July 2014.

with other facilities, including in the private sector. Accordingly, in 1998 the Commission proposed extending the directive to cover excluded sectors including doctors in training. The updated directive agreed on this basis in 2000[122] did extend the original directive to cover doctors in training but provided a specific further transitional period of up to eight years with higher limits on working time for doctors in training (an average of 58 hours a week, progressively falling to 52 hours a week). This again was in order to take account of the specific difficulties of health system organization, in particular put forward by the United Kingdom. These directives were then further amended and consolidated in 2003, with broadly the same provisions although with a cap on weekly working hours of 48 hours. The directive included similar derogations for longer working hours for doctors in training as the 2000 directive. It also allowed Member States to provide for exceptions allowing employees to choose to work longer hours if they wished, and for managers to be exempted from the cap.

Given the size of changes brought by the directive in comparison with the historical practice of doctors working well over 100 hours a week, it is perhaps not surprising that some doctors and managers were critical of the provisions to reduce working hours, arguing that these would reduce the scope for clinical training, and discounting the benefits to patients from fewer fatigue-related errors and to the long-term health of doctors themselves.[123] Indeed, it has taken considerable time and debate to arrive at models of care organization that reconcile these different objectives, and the issue is still debated. However, the criticisms that the EU working time legislation had been developed without taking account of its impact on health systems is more difficult to understand, given that this had been a central part of the European debate since the original directive in 1993, as is the general absence of engagement of health professionals from this debate until the stage of implementation of the 2003 directive in the mid-2000s. This seems to be another example where the wider health community did not understand or engage with the impact of Europe on health – perhaps because the formal basis of the working time directives was health and safety at work, rather than the article on public health, and discussion largely took place in employment-related forums rather than the Health Council, for example.

3.3.3   Social partners in EU law

As mentioned above, social policy also has a unique additional legislative route, which is by direct negotiation and agreement between management and union

---

122 European Parliament and Council (2000). Directive 2000/34/EC amending Council Directive 93/104/ EC concerning certain aspects of the organization of working time to cover sectors and activities excluded from that Directive. *Official Journal*, L 195:41–4.

123 Mossialos E et al. (eds). (2010). *Health systems governance in Europe: the role of EU law and policy.* Cambridge: Cambridge University Press.

representatives (aka social partners); these agreements can then be implemented into normal EU law by a Commission proposal and Council decision.[124] The only use of this procedure in healthcare was the directive on sharps, such as needles, which are a major health and safety issue in healthcare (*see* section 3.3.1).

3.3.4 Equalities and nondiscrimination

One key area where there are strong EU measures is that of nondiscrimination. Here the EU has strong powers to prohibit discrimination on six grounds – gender, racial or ethnic origin, religion or belief, disability, age, and sexual orientation[125] – and it has put in place wide-ranging legislation to combat discrimination on these grounds. The EU is also a signatory to the United Nations Convention on the Rights of Persons with Disabilities.[126] The United Nations Convention, intriguingly, defines people with disabilities as those "who have long-term physical, mental, intellectual or sensory impairments which in interaction with various barriers may hinder their full and effective participation in society on an equal basis with others".[127] People with chronic conditions could clearly be considered to fall within this definition (e.g. people needing dialysis, the provision of which prevents them from being able to keep a full-time job). However, patient groups have been reluctant to claim the label of disability, despite the strong EU legal protections that it brings – ill-health as such is not a protected ground of discrimination.

3.4 Consumer protection

Consumer protection in the European Union, like environmental protection and, to some extent, health, grew up in internal market law before becoming part of the treaties in 1992 at Maastricht. In other words, the 1992 appearance of consumer protection as its own treaty article (then Article 153, now Article 169) did not mean that it only became a concern then but rather that it became an additional treaty base useful for complementing or redirecting concerns to do with regulation of the internal market. The objectives of the EU on consumer protection include contributing to "the *health*, safety and economic interests of consumers" (emphasis added).[128] These objectives are principally achieved through internal market legislation, but internal market measures protecting the health of consumers (consumers being understood in EU law as anyone acting outside their trade or profession) can also be justified on the basis of the consumer

---

124 TFEU, Article 153. For more political background, *see* Johnson A. (2005). *European Welfare States and Supranational Governance of Social Policy*. London: Palgrave Macmillan, pp. 1–27.
125 TFEU, Articles 10 and 19.
126 European Commission (2010). *European disability strategy 2010–2020: a renewed commitment to a barrier-free Europe (COM(2010)636)*. Brussels: European Commission.
127 United Nations (2006). *Convention on the rights of persons with disabilities*. New York: United Nations.
128 TFEU, Article 169.

protection article with and using the ordinary legislative procedure on its treaty base. Examples include food safety, labelling and nutritional health claims. Organizationally, consumer protection was linked with public health to create DG SANCO under the Prodi Commission, but it was delinked and moved to the DG for Justice and Consumers (DG JUST) under the Juncker Commission.

The keystone of EU consumer protection law is found in two old directives. The Product Liability Directive of 1985 imposed strict liability on enterprises for harm to consumers from defective products, with the definition of a defect flowing from what consumers should be entitled to expect. The Unfair Terms in Consumer Contracts Directive of 1993 deems a contract unfair and not binding if it "causes a significant imbalance in the parties' rights and obligations arising under the contract, to the detriment of the consumer". There is a substantial focus on nondiscrimination, e.g. in the presence of a network of European Consumer Centres (ECC-net), which provide national contact points to explain consumer rights and assist with cross-border issues. Nowadays the rights of consumers include a minimum 14-day right to return a product and a two-year guarantee against faulty goods, using standards that include the claims made by suppliers.

Overall, the law is clear and has been interpreted by Member State and EU courts as giving consumers a right to redress for defective products and making unfair contracts nonbinding, taking into account the weaker position of consumers vis-à-vis business, which means that they should get more protection than businesses in commercial contracts. This is a potentially thoroughgoing agenda with implications for both healthcare services and for public health in general. It has had relatively little impact on healthcare services because most healthcare providers and professionals have clearly defined professional scope of practice and remedies exist for underperformance. It might be used more forcefully on the edges of the healthcare sector, e.g. with the regulation of vitamins, supplements and m-health such as fitness trackers. It might theoretically also be used on products with serious health consequences, such as alcohol or fast food, though that would take a major reorientation of the law. It is not clear that any such reorientation is coming. The Commission's last major strategic document was published in 2012[129] and is filled with the language and preoccupations of that era. While there are obvious industry lobbies, including healthcare lobbies, that would oppose a revival of the consumer protection agenda, it also has potential as a way for the EU to both promote health and make clear its contribution to health, while still operating within a clear treaty base and mandate to pursue the four freedoms.

---

129 COM/2012/0225 final. Communication from the Commission to the European Parliament, the Council, the Economic and Social Committee and the Committee of the Regions (2012). A European Consumer Agenda – Boosting confidence and growth.

Fig. 3.1   *Major causes of death by age group in the EU25*

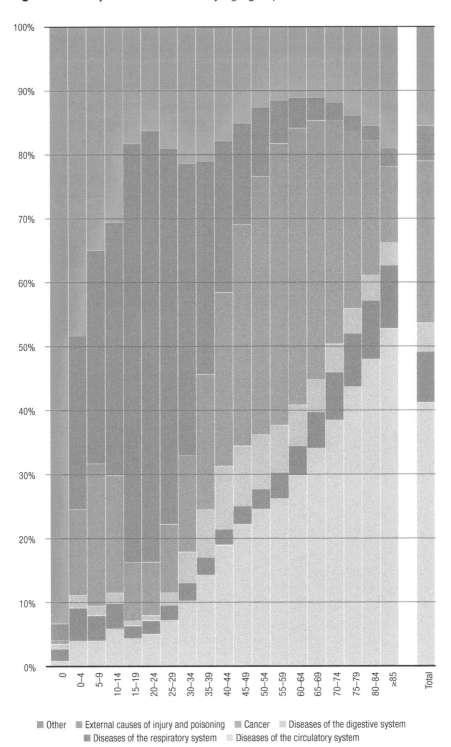

Other   External causes of injury and poisoning   Cancer   Diseases of the digestive system
Diseases of the respiratory system   Diseases of the circulatory system

3.5 Health systems values

What has the EU done to shape health systems thinking, or at least the impact of EU policies on health systems? The EU has produced a number of key statements that guide its policies and enable or constrain new initiatives. In healthcare, the 2006 statement on health systems values has helped to shape the place of health systems as a distinctive policy concern with shared moral values that should influence policy. The European Pillar of Social Rights covers a wide range of policies, most with health relevance, and also explicitly focuses on health systems values. Both help to influence broader EU policy such as the Semester by making it clear what values, besides fiscal sustainability, the Member States agreed. They are separate from the extensive law and policy discussed in chapter 4, the second face, which focus on healthcare providers and purchasers in the internal market rather than health *systems*.

3.5.1 2006 statement on health systems values

The 2006 *Council Conclusions on Common values and principles in European Union Health Systems*[130] is in part a creature of its time, reflecting a specific agreement by Member States under the UK presidency that contemporary efforts to incorporate healthcare into the general internal market for services (e.g. with the first proposed Services Directive) were inappropriate and did not reflect the core values of their healthcare systems. The existence of the statement undercut any new efforts to assimilate healthcare with the principles regulating other sectors and also shape broader discussions of health policy, including in the Semester.

3.5.2 Effective, accessible and resilient health systems

The next key statement of values and priorities came from the EPSCO Council in late 2013 Conclusions, and was followed by the Commission with a 2014 Communication.[131] The Council Conclusions were a wide-ranging statement of health values and priorities, and the value of health as a general European priority. It was, among other things, a response by health ministers to the reinforced fiscal governance system's inroads into health policy (see chapter 5), reiterating the importance of health and health systems and encouraging the EU in a supportive role. The Commission translated this request into the 2014 Communication. These two documents superseded the 2006 Council conclusions. It sets out three Commission goals in the area of health systems: "1. Strengthen the effectiveness of

---

130 Council Conclusions on Common values and principles in European Union Health Systems (2006/C 146/01).
131 Council conclusions on the "Reflection process on modern, responsive and sustainable health systems" Brussels, 10 December 2013; Commission Communication on effective, accessible and resilient health systems, April 2014 COM(2014) 215.

Box 3.5   *The European Pillar of Social Rights*

The Pillar of Social Rights builds upon 20 key principles, structured around three categories:

I. Equal opportunities and access to the labour market

II. Fair working conditions

III. Social protection and inclusion

I. Equal opportunities and access to the labour market

   1.   Education, training and lifelong learning

   2.   Gender equality

   3.   Equal opportunities

   4.   Active support to employment

II. Fair working conditions

   5.   Secure and adaptable employment

   6.   Wages

   7.   Information about employment conditions and protection in case of dismissals

   8.   Social dialogue and involvement of workers

   9.   Work–life balance

  10. Healthy, safe and well-adapted work environment and data protection

III. Social protection and inclusion

  11. Childcare and support to children

  12. Social protection

  13. Unemployment benefits

  14. Minimum income

  15. Old age income and pensions

  16. Healthcare

  17. Inclusion of people with disabilities

  18. Long-term care

  19. Housing and assistance for the homeless

  20. Access to essential services

health systems 2. Increase the accessibility of healthcare 3. Improve the resilience of health systems." While many of the actions necessary to achieve this are by design to be taken at the member state level, the Communication lists a variety of EU actions from Health Systems Performance Assessment (HSPA) to Health Technology Assessment (HTA) that contribute to member states' policies and effectiveness. Most of the topics covered by this Communication are discussed throughout chapter 3 and in section 4.3.

3.5.3 The European Pillar of Social Rights

The European Pillar of Social Rights (EPSR) was declared by the Council, Parliament and European Commission in 2017.[132] It has twenty principles – twenty rights – in the categories of "Equal opportunities and access to the labour market", "Fair working conditions" and "Social protection and inclusion".

As ever with EU health policy, it is tempting to turn directly to the category of "social protection and inclusion" and look for the healthcare principle, but almost all of these rights affect health and many can be affected by healthcare systems. Homelessness, for example, is both a major public health problem (a short period of homelessness can have lasting and diverse negative health effects) and is often caused by failures in healthcare, especially to do with mental health treatment. "Work–life balance" is categorized as being about "fair working conditions", but the evidence is impressive that supporting parents in their work reaps health benefits for everybody in the family. "Fair working conditions" also includes an explicit right to a healthy workplace, for workplaces and work practices are indeed a key source of ill- or good health and employers do not always provide them without regulation. "Gender equality", for a third example, is in "Equal opportunities and access to the labour market" but is a key determinant of the well-being and health of all genders.

That said, there is healthcare content, the simple: "Everyone has the right to timely access to affordable, preventive and curative health care of good quality." It is complemented by a commitment to long-term care: "Everyone has the right to affordable long-term care services of good quality, in particular home-care and community-based services." It is worth underlining that the EPSR is, by the standards of most political systems, both ambitious and concrete. Even if its main effect is to limit contradictory policy initiatives within the EU and empower advocates within the Member States, that is significant, and its ambitions are impressive.[133]

3.5.4 Charter of Fundamental Rights

The Charter of Fundamental Rights became part of EU constitutional law when the Lisbon Treaty entered into force in 2009. It brings together rights that had been in EU law, including the Social Charter, and in member state constitutional law. It was drafted and proclaimed by the EU institutions in 2000, and then

---

132 European Commission. Proclamation of the European Pillar of Social Rights. 16 November 2017. Brussels: European Commission.
133 For the political background of the EPSR, as a case study in how the EU approach to social policy has changed in the last decade, *see* Sabato S, Vanhercke B (2017). Towards a European Pillar of Social Rights: from a preliminary outline to a Commission Recommendation, in B Vanhercke, S Sabato and D Bourget, eds. *Social policy in the European Union: state of play*, pp. 73–96.

was incorporated into the Lisbon Treaty. The rights listed in the Charter are fundamental and justiciable under EU law, and applies to infringements of rights by EU law or member states implementing EU law. It incorporates the separate European Convention on Human Rights, which is not EU law.

3.6 Health policy processes

Health, in part because the Article 168 treaty base is so limited, has been the scene of quite a lot of experimentation in newer forms of governance that seek to coordinate and change policy through means other than hard law. This section presents some of the key initiatives intended to improve health policies and systems, which means that it does not cover measures built primarily out of internal market law. Those are discussed in chapter 4. In particular, Directive 2011/24/EU on Patients' Rights in Cross-Border Healthcare was a response to Member State and European courts' application of internal market law to healthcare, discussed in section 4.3.1. It emerged from debates about the proper application of internal market law even if by the end the Directive recognized the specificity of health thanks to interventions such as the 2006 Council Conclusions (see section 1.5). It became the basis for initiatives in areas such as e-Health, and healthcare quality that are discussed in sections 4.3.3–5. It is not to be confused with the European Convention on Human Rights, which is a separate Council of Europe instrument, but all of which is incorporated into the Charter of Fundamental Rights. The Fundamental Rights Agency advises on Charter issues.

Article 35, reproduced in the Appendix, specifically states a right to health care and health protection. Other articles incorporate health, e.g. Article 31 specifies a right to healthy working conditions.

3.6.1   State of health in the EU cycle

Developed in cooperation with the Organisation for Economic Co-operation and Development (OECD) and the European Observatory on Health Systems and Policies, *State of Health in the EU* is a two-year initiative undertaken by the European Commission that aims to provide health policy-makers and other relevant actors with comparative data into health systems in EU countries.[134]

Launched in 2016, the two-year *State of Health in the EU* cycle consists of four stages. The first began with the publication of *Health at a Glance: Europe*, a comparative overview of EU health systems. This 2018 joint report of the European Commission and the OECD found that the steady increase of life

---

134 European Commission. State of Health in the EU. Available at: https://ec.europa.eu/health/state/ summary_en.

expectancy in Europe has slowed down, and that health disparities according to sex and socioeconomic status persist both within and between EU Member States.[135] The report also called for improving mental health, after 84 000 people died of the consequences of mental illness in 2015, and the total cost arising from lack of or undertreatment amounts to €600 billion per year. It also called for ensuring universal access to care, addressing risk factors such as smoking and drinking, and strengthening the resilience of health systems through, for instance, the pricing of pharmaceutical drugs through health technology assessment.

The second step in the cycle is the periodical publication of *Country Health Profiles* for all EU Member States. This joint publication of the European Commission, the OECD and the European Observatory on Health Systems and Policies gives a snapshot of each country's population's state of health and key risk factors, along with an analysis of each health system's performance in terms of effectiveness, accessibility and resilience. The third step is the publication of a Companion Report, to be released alongside the Country Health Profiles, which links common policy priorities across EU Member States. Finally, when the project reaches the end of the two-year cycle, health authorities will be able to request voluntary exchanges with the experts behind the studies to discuss potential policy responses. This is not just an academic exercise. It substantially informs the European Semester (chapter 5, e.g. Box 5.2).

3.6.2 Health programme

A core tool for the EU's specific action on health has been financing collaborative projects on health. This started as a series of topic-specific programmes (e.g. on cancer) before being integrated into a single funding programme for health. The third health programme[136] finances a range of collaborative projects across Europe around the three broad headings of health threats, health determinants and health information. However, the key point about the programme is its size, or rather lack of it; a budget of around €46 million a year equates to 0.000058% of publicly funded health expenditure in the EU,[137] or around one half of one millionth part. Even if compared with only the preventive part of national expenditure (around 3%), the programme's resources remain relatively

---

135 European Commission (2018). Press release: State of Health in the EU: more protection and prevention for longer and healthier lives. Brussels, European Commission, 22 November 2018.

136 European Parliament and Council (2014). Regulation (EU) No. 282/2014 on the establishment of a third programme for the European Union's action in the field of health (2014–2020). *Official Journal*, 86:1–13; in general, *see* European Commission (2014). Health programme. Luxembourg: Publications Office of the European Union. Available at: http://ec.europa.eu/health/programme/policy/index_en.htm, accessed 4 July 2014.

137 Source for comparison figure of total public health expenditure: OECD (2012). *Health at a glance: Europe 2012*. Paris: Organisation for Economic Co-operation and Development; source for comparison figure of total EU GDP (2010 figure): European Commission (2014). *Eurostat statistics*. Brussels: Eurostat. Available at: http://epp.eurostat.ec.europa.eu/portal/page/portal/eurostat/home/, accessed 4 July 2014.

tiny. This small sum means that the EU cannot provide most of what a health system does; it does not, and will never, have enough money to do so, and it will always be engaged in supplementary actions.

Despite this relative lack of resources, the health programme has been effective in sharing knowledge, supporting collaborations between countries and generating comparable data for benchmarking; such European projects have changed the direction of entire national health systems, such as in the case of cancer, by highlighting comparisons.[138] They show a strong bias towards supporting capacity building, often among EU-level groups such as the Association of Schools of Public Health of the European Region, the European Federation of Associations of Dietitians, and conferences or research projects intended to identify and promote good practice. A mid-term evaluation found that the health programme excelled in promoting networking but appeared to distribute its projects rather thinly.[139] Nevertheless, this limited volume of resources inevitably affects the scope for EU-financed action on health.

The Commission has proposed a major change for the future. For the upcoming period of the Multi-annual Financial Framework (2021–2027), the Commission has proposed ending the health programme as a separate funding stream and instead integrating it within the European Social Fund Plus (ESF+) as part of the European Structural and Investment Funds. This is more than an administrative reorganization; rather, it is likely to represent a fundamental shift in the EU's support for health. On the one hand, it means that health objectives are formally and specifically included in the proposed ESF+, as regards both public health and health systems, which potentially marks a very substantial increase in the resources available for health at EU level. On the other hand, the actual amount of money specifically allocated to health is around €30m *less* than in the previous programming period, and the degree of influence of health actors on how this money is spent is likely to be much reduced. Although the Commission proposes mechanisms for "consultation" of health authorities, the actual decision-making regarding funding would be made through the processes for the ESF+ as a whole.[140] At the time of writing, these proposals are still being considered by the Council and the new Parliament; their exact impact on the EU's financial support for health will depend on how the tensions described above are addressed.

138 Briatte F (2013). "The politics of European public health data", in Greer SL & Kurzer P (eds.). *European Union public health policies: regional and global perspectives*. Abingdon: Routledge, pp. 51–63.

139 Public Health and Impact Assessment Consortium (2011). *Mid-term evaluation of the health programme (2008–2013)*. Bologna: Public Health and Impact Assessment Consortium. Available at: http://ec.europa.eu/health/programme/docs/mthp_final_report_oct2011_en.pdf accessed 4 July 2014.

140 *See* COM(2018)382. Proposal for a Regulation of the European Parliament and of the Council on the European Social Fund Plus (ESF+), 30 May 2018.

3.6.3 Expert Group in Health System Performance Assessment

Given the increased interest in monitoring EU Member States' health systems and assessing their comparative performance, also in the context of the European Semester, the Commission in 2014 set up an Expert Group on Health Systems Performance Assessment (HSPA), consisting of representatives from all EU Member States (and Norway). The aim was to develop a common understanding on HSPA approaches, tools and methodologies, through sharing national experiences in this field. Experts from WHO, OECD and the European Observatory on Health Systems and Policies provide additional support and advice. Work so far has focused on how to assess performance in specific domains including quality, efficiency, primary care, integrated care and resilience.

3.6.4 Expert Panel on Effective Ways of Investing in Health

To ensure timely, scientific, non-binding advice on strategically relevant health matters, the European Commission set up in 2012 a multidisciplinary independent Expert Panel on Effective Ways of Investing in Health. Its overall aim is to make scientific contributions to the effectiveness, accessibility and resilience of European health systems.[141] At the same time, the work of the panel acknowledges the contribution of public health and health systems to health and wealth in the European Union. This contrasts with mere cost-containment or austerity policies as promoted by other Directorates-general. The panel consists of 14 members who serve a three-year term. The panel has produced continuously a large number of opinions concerning, for example, digital transformation, cross-border care and vaccination.[142]

3.6.5 The EU Health Policy Forum

The EU Health Policy Platform is a consultation mechanism funded by the Health Programme, the largest and one of a long series of institutionalized consultative mechanisms organized by the health DG. It is an open platform, with over 5 000 members at the time of writing, ranging from the Brewers of Europe and the European Association of Sugar Manufacturers to the Irish Cancer Society and the Caritas of the Diocese of Coimbra in Portugal (to select from the 60 organizations attending its November 2018 meeting). Membership and engagement reflect an interest in health policy, not a stance, as seen in the presence of industry. It has a variety of activities, including an annual meeting, an award, and thematic groups that can formulate agendas to develop over a year, with participation voluntary and a presentation at the annual meeting. As with most of these consultative

---

141 Available at: https://ec.europa.eu/health/expert_panel/sites/expertpanel/files/rules_of_procedure_en.pdf.
142 All opinions are available online at: https://ec.europa.eu/health/expert_panel/home_en.

groups, it is a way for stakeholders, including poorly resourced ones, to maintain some contact with the Commission and each other and remain informed, and for the Commission to validate thinking and test out support for different policy ideas. Its importance varies with the importance the Commission assigns to it, which participants can easily monitor by, for example, seeing who participates from the Commission. It diffuses technical and political information, formally and informally, but its impact on policy or its members is unclear.

3.6.6 The Working Party on Public Health at the Senior Level

The Working Party on Public Health at the Senior Level is a Council working group which can provide input on behalf of ministers on a wide range of topics. In the Semester it has a role in consultation on health recommendations. As a Council formation, its importance can vary with the presidency; for example, the 2018 Austrian presidency tended to call meetings only at the attaché level.

3.7   Global health and international engagement

The European Union is a major global health actor and is deeply engaged in complex relationships with many countries. This is a major policy area with high stakes and large sums of money involved, and we can give only a brief account here of its health dimensions.

3.7.1   European neighbourhood policies

"Neighbourhood policies" refer to policies directed at the EU's close southern and eastern neighbours. To the south, that means Algeria, Egypt, Israel, Jordan, Lebanon, Libya, Morocco, Palestine, Syria and Tunisia. To the east, that means Armenia, Azerbaijan, Belarus, Georgia, Moldova and Ukraine. As the list makes clear, Europe lives in a complex and diverse neighbourhood, and it is hard to develop policies for relations with these countries as a group. Tunisia and Libya, or Belarus and Ukraine, are in quite different situations with quite different orientations towards Europe.

Two large states in the neighbourhood are not covered by "neighbourhood" policies. Russia participates in some neighbourhood policies but generally prefers to deal bilaterally with EU Member States, and, if it deals with the EU, is reluctant to be clustered with smaller post-Soviet states. In the past the Russian Federation and some of its regional governments did participate in some surveillance and other networks, e.g. the communicable disease surveillance joint action EPINORTH (which ended in 2012). Given that managing tensions with Russia is more of a priority than closer integration at the moment, it is not reasonable to expect much more.

Turkey has been in a customs union with the EU since 1995 and a candidate Member State with theoretically ongoing accession negotiations, though the negotiations are frozen on a variety of grounds (including democratic backsliding and Cyprus, as well as the manifest hostility of a number of Member States to Turkish accession). They are unlikely to restart soon.

Other south-east European non-Member States – Albania, Bosnia and Herzegovina, Kosovo,[143] Montenegro, North Macedonia and Serbia – are also dealt with as enlargement candidates rather than neighbours. These relations are closer, and aid to those countries travels through different financial instruments. As with Turkey, being a candidate for EU enlargement implies nothing about the actual probability of accession in the near future, and some of these states are unlikely to join the EU very soon.

Issues of migration and security, not health, dominate relations to the south,[144] and so the health dimensions of these relations are ones that emerge from a policy focused on migration. Turkey is programmed to receive €6 billion through a programme called the EU Facility for Turkey by the end of 2020 (two two-year programmes of €3 billion each). The explicit goal of this programme is to allow Turkey to manage flows of refugees who would otherwise attempt to enter the EU. It was created in 2016 and was substantially responsible for the end of 2015's highly controversial refugee movements. It is linked with discussions of liberalizing EU visas for Turkish citizens. Libya, likewise, is a failed state and a jumping-off point for many refugees and undocumented migrants in the extremely dangerous sea crossing to Europe. EU interests in a stable Libya that can control both outbound migratory flows and the organized crime associated with undocumented migration have not been easy to achieve.

In this broader context, the European Neighbourhood Policy has changed quickly. It is, through 2020, financed through the European Neighbourhood Instrument (ENI), which provides a policy framework and budget. Most of what it involves is bilateral cooperation, given the diverse political difficulties in the region. It also supports regional groupings such as the Eastern Partnership and Union for the Mediterranean.

The EU suspended all bilateral cooperation with the Syrian government in 2011. The EU Regional Trust Fund in Response to the Syrian Crisis supports refugees

---

143 Note that the designation of Kosovo is without prejudice to positions of status, and in line with the United Nations Security Council Resolution 1244/99, and the International Court of Justice opinion on the Kosovo declaration of independence.
144 Del Sarto RA, Steindler C (2015). Uncertainties at the European Union's southern borders: actors, policies, and legal frameworks. *European Security*, 24(3):369–80.

from Syria and locals affected by the refugee flows and crisis in Lebanon, Egypt, Turkey, Jordan, Iraq and the Western Balkans. Its health dimension, which complements other aspects of the programme such as education, water and sanitation, supports primary care and access to medicines and targets for over a million refugees.

The lead DGs for neighbourhood issues are, unsurprisingly, DG NEAR (DG European Neighbourhood Policy and Enlargement Negotiations) and to a lesser extent DG ECHO (Humanitarian Aid and Civil Protection) and the European External Action Service, which is not part of the Commission and responds to the EU's High Representative of the Union for Foreign Affairs and Security Policy, Federica Mogherini until 2019 and Josep Borrell from 2019.

Health is not one of the four neighborhood policy priority areas, which have been recast around governance, economic and social development, security and cooperation against radicalization, and migration and mobility. It is not even in the second tier of priorities around energy security and climate action. There are health projects being funded, but primarily as other topics. This is in contrast to the older iterations of the ENP, which pre-dated many of the current security concerns arising both east and south of the EU and which had more cooperative work on topics such as surveillance, phytosanitary standards and veterinary health. There is a larger component of health-related EU assistance and cooperation with the accession candidate states, particularly those in the Balkans.

3.7.2   Global health: European development aid

The EU is the world's largest donor and health is a major component of European aid. We can only give a very abbreviated account of this complex world in which the EU is a very important actor.

Broadly, aid comes in two categories: relief and development. Relief is aid in response to particular humanitarian situations such as war, natural disasters, displacement of peoples, and famine. Development aid is geared towards longer-term assistance in areas such as education, health and economic development. The leading DG for development is DG DEVCO, the Directorate-General for International Cooperation and Development. For humanitarian crises and relief, the lead DG is DG ECHO, the DG for Humanitarian Aid and Civil Protection. In relief, the EU provides aid and also operates RescEU, the EU Civil Protection Mechanism (*see* section 3.1.4) which assists victims of natural or human-caused disasters globally and, more recently, in the EU.

EU development aid touches on many areas of health. Health priorities[145] range from strengthening health systems to assistance with International Health Regulation implementation to contributions to the Global Fund to Fight AIDS, Tuberculosis and Malaria. It provided around €2 billion annually of total development in the budget ending in 2020. Climate finance and sustainable growth are the key EU priorities, though the EU endorses all of the SDGs in its foreign aid. Discussions surrounding the post-2020 budget have involved proposals for both expansion and greater flexibility in the EU's ability to direct aid.

According to the OECD, the EU spent around €1 billion on global health in 2016 (the last year for which data are available), about 5% of its total health expenditures. This is partly because the EU negotiates aid priorities with each recipient state, and only fifteen countries had requested it for that aid budget period. The 2017 "EU consensus on development" calls for the EU to spend 20% of aid on health and social inclusion.[146] That said, the 5% probably undercounts the contribution to EU development aid to health, since aid in areas such as nutrition and literacy almost certainly contributes to better health.

The foundation of the EU approach as of now dates to a Commission Communication endorsed by the Council in 2010.[147] It identifies as key challenges the achievement of universal health coverage (UHC), policy coherence ("health policy can not be handled in isolation") and knowledge ("research that benefits all"). It should "apply the common values and principles of solidarity towards equitable and universal coverage of quality health services in all external and internal policies and actions", including inclusiveness with regards to stakeholders within and across countries.

3.7.3   Global health voice

The same 2010 Communication and Council Conclusions[148] that underpin the EU's development aid also encourage the EU to develop its own policy coherence among different elements of the EU that affect global health, including trade policy, health policy, civil protection policy and development aid. It also calls on

---

145 https://ec.europa.eu/europeaid/sectors/human-development/health_en.

146 The New European Consensus on Development, 'Our World, Our Dignity, Our Future', joint statement by the Council and the Representatives of the Governments of the Member States meeting within the Council, the European Parliament and the European Commission. Available at: https://ec.europa.eu/europeaid/sites/devco/files/european-consensus-on-development-final-20170626_en.pdf.

147 COM(2010)128 final. Communication from the Commission to the Council, the European Parliament, the European Economic and Social Committee and the Committee of the Regions. The EU Role in Global Health and Council conclusions on the EU role in Global Health. 3011th Foreign Affairs Council meeting, Brussels, 10 May 2010.

148 COM(2010)128 final. Communication from the Commission to the Council, the European Parliament, the European Economic and Social Committee and the Committee of the Regions. The EU Role in Global Health and Council conclusions on the EU role in Global Health. 3011th Foreign Affairs Council meeting, Brussels, 10 May 2010.

EU institutions and Member States to support the WHO, including a reduction in earmarked funding.[149]

3.8 Research

Research has long been a major EU priority, with clear potential added-value from collaboration between scientists across Europe, with the largest part of the EU budget after the Common Agricultural Policy and the structural funds. In general, research policy anywhere has some combination of three points of focus: it can be industrial policy (promoting industry and economic growth), science policy (promoting basic research, science infrastructure and knowledge), or substantive (focused on generating knowledge about a particular topic, such as climate change or health). EU research policy has never been primarily a science policy and has always had a strong industrial policy component. In the last decade in particular, it has been especially focused on industrial policy objectives.[150]

Health has been a major priority within that, and the EU has funded thousands of health-related research projects.[151] Despite the collective challenges facing the EU in terms of public health and health systems, described above, health-related research has tended to avoid these topics, primarily funding biomedical research of more general application instead.[152]

This may change in the coming decades. The EU's research programme Horizon 2020[153] has a broader focus than in the past on "health, demographic change and well-being". Under Horizon 2020, health research fields include health, environment and lifestyle, mental health, foresight, health systems and services, research for maternal and child health, and global health, although in practice the biomedical approach has remained central. The increased EU focus on broader health system issues, for example the recommendations being made by the EU to Member States about health system reform through the processes of the European Semester, is likely to increase pressure to shift the focus of the EU's funding to more relevant research in the years to come. The potential of the health systems of the Member States to learn from each other has been much

---

149 For a broader and more reflective analysis, see Hervey TK (2017). "The EU's (emergent) global health law and policy", in Hervey TK, Young C & Bishop L (eds.). *Research Handbook on EU Law and Policy*. Cheltenham: Edward Elgar Publishing, pp. 453–78.

150 Greer SL, Kuhlmann E (2019). "Health and Education Policy: Labour Markets, Qualifications, and the Struggle over Standards", in St John SK & Murphy M (eds.). *Education and Public Policy in the European Union*. London: Palgrave Macmillan, pp. 67–88.

151 Charlesworth K et al. (2011). Health research in the European Union: over-controlled but under-measured? *European Journal of Public Health*, 21(4):404–6.

152 Walshe K et al. (2013). Health systems and policy research in Europe: Horizon 2020. *Lancet*, 382(9893):668–9.

153 European Parliament and Council (2013). Regulation (EU) No. 1291/2013 establishing Horizon 2020 – the framework programme for research and innovation (2014–2020) – and repealing Decision No. 1982/2006/EC. *Official Journal*, L 347:104.

discussed in principle, but has proved remarkably hard to do in practice. The TO-REACH project, for example, has aimed to address this by providing a basis for a joint European research programme on health services and systems. Its proposed Strategic Research Agenda outlines a European strategy to advance our knowledge and understanding of the adoption, implementation and potential scale-up of service and policy innovations and their translation to other settings within and across countries. Given the shared challenges facing European health systems, realizing the potential of learning and working together should become an increasingly central part of European health research.

Of course, the EU's funding for research is only a small part of total public funding for research in the EU. The bulk of funding comes from national governments, directly or through higher education, and through industry (mostly for more applied technology). National, regional and private strategies are not coordinated, and many EU countries have lacked overall strategies for health research.[154] Consequently part of the EU's role has become not only to fund research but also to help to coordinate European funding of research more generally to maximize effectiveness and avoid duplication. This has been the case through examples of "joint programming initiatives", including on the specific health topics of Alzheimer's disease and other neurodegenerative diseases, healthy diet and physical activity, antimicrobial resistance and the implications of demographic change.[155] There is, as yet, no more general strategy for coordination of research across Europe in relation to the challenges faced by health systems; again, this may emerge onto the agenda in the coming years with the increasing policy focus on these questions.[156]

3.9 Conclusion

The pioneering work of the Commission on Social Determinants of Health led by Professor Sir Michael Marmot underlined the importance of social factors for health. This, however, is the area where the "constitutional asymmetry" of the EU in regard to health is clearest. While the EU has significant action on some of the social determinants that the Commission identified (in particular working conditions, as discussed in section 3.2.5, and more general protection of employment conditions), questions of income, tax, social protection and the extent of solidarity within societies are some of the core areas reserved by Member States for national action rather than being EU responsibilities. The

---

154 Grimaud O, McCarthy M, Conceicao C (2013). Strategies for public health research in European Union countries. *European Journal of Public Health*, 23(suppl 2):35–8.

155 European Commission. *Joint programming initiatives*. Brussels: European Commission. Available at: http://ec.europa.eu/research/era/joint-programming-initiatives_en.html, accessed 4 July 2014.

156 Walshe K et al. (2013). Health systems and policy research in Europe: Horizon 2020. *Lancet*, 382(9893):668–9.

powers of the EU to create an internal market have knock-on consequences (shifting employment in a particular profession from one country to another, for example). The social protection systems to ensure support such as unemployment protection and retraining, nevertheless, are a national responsibility. There is potential support from sources such as the European Social Fund, but this is, of course, relatively marginal in comparison with the cost of social protection systems overall.

This is not to say that the EU has been inactive. The EU has focused attention on issues such as access for all to education, social protection and healthcare; creating jobs and equal opportunities; and promoting social inclusion; it has also specifically highlighted issues of health inequalities. A Charter of Fundamental Rights of the European Union has also been adopted, which includes a range of social provisions (see Appendix). The problem is that the principal tools to meet these objectives and rights, both legislative and overwhelmingly financial, are at national level, not European.

The first face of European Union health policy is shaped by the constitutional asymmetry of the EU and by its nature as a primarily regulatory state, as discussed in chapter 1. *Constitutional asymmetry* means that positive action such as health systems strengthening is limited by the difficulty of the EU legislative process, by subsidiarity as both a principle and an objective of many Member States, and by the EU budget, which is kept small. By contrast, action to remove Member State policies in the name of the internal market – the second face and focus of the next chapter – has stronger legal bases and benefits from the large and highly developed EU legal system. The EU's reliance on *regulation* as its key policy tool, meanwhile, means that its greatest health effects are through law and regulation rather than through expenditure, and its effects via expenditure are often by shaping agendas, norms and networks rather than by actively financing activities. Thus the most effective and consequential EU health policies, viewed in the round, are regulatory, whether on food safety, environmental protection or the internal market.

Chapter 4

The EU market shaping health

The second face of the EU in health policy is its action in the internal market. The internal market builds on the most powerful treaty bases and jurisprudence in the EU, and core legal concepts such as nondiscrimination, proportionality and mutual recognition (Box 2.2) facilitate its construction. The "four freedoms" in the internal market are the freedom of movement of goods, services, people and capital. The first three have all been turned into consequential policies on health and health systems. The last affects health indirectly, through shaping economies and providing the basis for fiscal governance. It thereby is at the root of the fiscal governance discussed in chapter 5.

The internal market built around the four freedoms is not always the basis of law and legislation that has been helpful to health and health systems. But it is worth remembering that a great deal of useful policy has been made on internal market treaty bases, often well beyond what is warranted by more apparently relevant treaty articles (HTA, for example, is a health policy on internal market treaty bases, as was environmental or consumer protection policy until 1992). What the second face does, however, is limit the policy instruments to law and regulation with some plausible connection to the market. In other words, the second face is about deregulation at the Member State level and reregulation at the EU level. The EU's greatest powers are legal and regulatory, and they mostly grow from internal market bases. Hence the importance of the EU's second face.

4.1 Goods

Health-related products are a major part of the internal market and have become one of the most European of sectors, with highly detailed European requirements governing them. Health has to be ensured for all products, whether they are specifically related to health or not, and this has been reflected in the wider rules for products within the EU.

4.1.1   Pharmaceuticals

Since 1965[1] the EU has been steadily harmonizing the rules governing the requirements to allow sale of medicinal products in the EU, to the extent where this is now one of the most regulated sectors of the European market.[2] Initially focused on setting common standards for national licensing bodies, the EU now has different options for licensing pharmaceuticals at either national or European level. The "centralized" procedure works with one single application for a licence, which is then valid for the entire EU; this route is compulsory for some product types, in particular those derived from biotechnology, and for those containing a new active substance licensed after May 2004 and intended to treat the priority conditions of HIV/AIDS, cancer, neurodegenerative diseases or diabetes. Otherwise, applications can be made to individual national authorities, with an approval granted by one national regulator then being recognized by others as and when applications are made to other countries. The European processes are run by one of the major health-related European agencies, the European Medicines Agency (EMA),[3] originally based in London and relocated to Amsterdam in 2019. The EMA also oversees the systems for monitoring any problems that may become apparent with medicines after they are licensed (the pharmacovigilance system).

The licensing process for pharmaceuticals is lengthy, with a sequence of three phases of clinical trials required before licensing in order to progressively provide the data necessary about the safety and efficacy of the product for the application to be evaluated.[4] The conduct of clinical trials is itself regulated at EU level,[5] although this has been controversial, with debate about whether the requirements imposed are too onerous, in particular for non-commercial applicants. Following pressure from patient groups, information about clinical trials is available through a database at the European level.[6]

---

1   European Council (1995). *Directive 65/65/EEC of 26 January 1965 on the approximation of provisions laid down by law, regulation or administrative action relating to medicinal products.* Brussels: European Commission.

2   Principally governed by Directive 2001/83/EC and Regulation (EC) No. 726/2004; see also Hauray B (2006). *L'Europe Du Médicament: Politique – Expertise – Intérêts Privés.* Paris: Presses de Sciences; Permanand G (2006). *EU pharmaceutical regulation: the politics of policy-making.* Manchester: Manchester University Press.

3   European Medicines Agency [web site]: http://www.ema.europa.eu/ema/.

4   World Health Organization (2014). *International clinical trials registry platform.* Geneva: World Health Organization. Available at: http://www.who.int/ictrp/glossary/en/index.html for more information about clinical trials, accessed 4 July 2014.

5   European Parliament and Council (2001). Directive 2001/20/EC on the approximation of the laws, regulations and administrative provisions of the Member States relating to the implementation of good clinical practice in the conduct of clinical trials on medicinal products for human use. *Official Journal*, L 121:34.

6   European Medicines Agency (2014). *EU clinical trials register.* Brussels: European Medicines Agency. Available at: https://www.clinicaltrialsregister.eu/ctr-search/search, accessed 4 July 2014.

> **Box 4.1**   *International dimensions of pharmaceuticals policy*
>
> Pharmaceutical supply chains are global, which means that detailed regulation of production and logistics is necessary to ensure quality and prevent fraud. The EU has signed mutual recognition pacts with regard to Good Manufacturing Practice with Australia, Canada, Japan, New Zealand, Switzerland, and the US as well as a similar agreement with Israel. EMA and the Commission also participate in international networks of regulators who focus on developing standards and identifying problems in regulation. Challenges remain in agreeing standards and their enforcement with regulators in China and India, both of which have large industries, and there are cooperative instruments to that end. Pharmaceuticals are also covered by trade agreements (see section 4.7) and enforcement of intellectual property law.[a] In all of these fields, the EU is one of the key forces shaping global standards and regulatory procedures within its trading partners.
>
> ----
>
> [a]   Massard da Fonseca E. "Intellectual property enforcement in the European Union" 126-138 in Greer SL and Kurzer P, eds. (2013) *European Union Public Health Policy*. Abingdon: Routledge.

The lengthy process that is required before authorization creates a different challenge, which is that companies developing new drugs have a period of several years between when they patent their potential products and when they are actually licensed and can be sold. Because of this, pharmaceutical products in the EU can have an extension of up to five years on top of the normal 20-year patent protection period.[7] The EU has also attempted to promote the development of drugs for rare diseases ("orphan drugs") through similar mechanisms, providing orphan medicines with ten years of market exclusivity after they are licensed.[8]

So far the regulatory regime resembles that of the world's other major pharmaceutical market, the United States. However, once we come to the stage of pricing, marketing and availability of pharmaceuticals, the EU looks very different. This is because, unlike the United States, more than half of pharmaceuticals are paid for by public funds, not privately, and the price of medicines and other healthcare products varies substantially between different EU countries, including as a result of specific national regulation.[9] Therefore, although the EU has a reasonably unified market access regime, its pricing models and markets remain fragmented between the Member States. They take quite different approaches and thereby produce the issue of "parallel trade" in pharmaceuticals that exploits interstate price differentials. The most that the EU has agreed on with regard to pricing is that the different regimes for pricing should at least be transparent in terms of

----

7   European Parliament and Council (2009). Regulation (EC) No. 469/2009 of 6 May 2009 concerning the supplementary protection certificate for medicinal products. *Official Journal*, L 152:1.

8   European Parliament and Council (2000). Regulation (EC) No. 141/2000 of 16 December 1999 on orphan medicinal products. *Official Journal*, L 18:1.

9   Ess SM, Schneeweiss S, Szucs TD (2003). European healthcare policies for controlling drug expenditure. *Pharmacoeconomics*, 21(2):89–103; Leopold C et al. (2012). Impact of external price referencing on medicine prices: a price comparison among 14 European countries. *Southern Medical Review*, 5(2):34.

providing information about the decisions they make, and they should do so within a reasonable time.[10] The actual transparency afforded by the Transparency Directive is by now minimal at best, since undisclosed rebates make published prices uninformative.

Within this picture of a fragmented market for pharmaceuticals, however, there are some areas of European consensus, the principal one being the horror with which European regulators (in particular in the European Parliament) view the widespread direct marketing of pharmaceuticals to consumers in the United States. Such direct-to-consumer advertising for prescription pharmaceuticals remains prohibited in Europe. Articles 86 to 100 of Directive 2001/83/EC on the Community code relating to medicinal products for human use[11] contain the general principles governing the advertising of drugs in the European Union. There is much ongoing debate about how to reconcile this with the recognized value to patients of having access to accurate information about pharmaceuticals and questions about which sources are likeliest to provide such information.[12] Efforts to liberalize direct-to-consumer 'information" launched in 2008 were withdrawn in 2014 after it became clear that the proposal would not pass.[13]

4.1.2　Medical devices

If regulation of pharmaceuticals is at one end of a scale (with strict scrutiny of detailed trials before products can be marketed) and the general EU approach for product safety is at the other end (with it being primarily up to manufacturers to ensure the safety of their own products), regulation of medical devices is somewhere in the middle.[14] While the relevant EU legislation has some requirements for initial scrutiny, these are lighter than for pharmaceutical products. Moreover, whereas licensing of pharmaceutical products is undertaken by public bodies (EMA and national agencies), the scrutiny of medical devices is undertaken by private companies that have been designated as "Notified Bodies"

10　European Commission (1989). Transparency Directive 89/105/EEC: transparency of measures relating to pricing and reimbursement of medicinal products. *Official Journal*, L 40:8.

11　Directive 2001/83/EC of the European Parliament and of the Council of 6 November 2001 on the Community code relating to medicinal products for human use.

12　*See* European Parliament (2008). *Medicinal products for human use: information on products subject to medical prescription*. Luxembourg: Publications Office of the European Union. Available at: http://www.europarl.europa.eu/oeil/popups/ficheprocedure.do?reference=2008/0256(COD)&l=en, accessed 14 July 2014.

13　For an illuminating account with regard to EU policy-making in this and other sectors, *see* Passarani I (2019). "Role of Evidence in the Formulation of European Public Health Policies". PhD thesis, Maastricht University.

14　A good account of the background can be found in Hancher L, Sauter W (2012). EU competition and internal market law in the health care sector. Oxford: Oxford University Press.

(NBs) by the competent authority of the Member State in question. There are around 60 such NBs in Europe.[15]

The requirements for marketing medical devices in the EU vary according to the level of risk that different medical products represent. At the low-risk end (class I devices), manufacturers themselves may simply declare that the products meet relevant standards. At the high-risk end (class III devices), NBs must be involved throughout their design and manufacture.[16] However, again unlike pharmaceuticals (and unlike the regulatory regime for medical devices in the United States), medical devices are not evaluated for their safety and effectiveness; rather, a narrower assessment is made of their safety and whether they function as intended. In practical terms, this means that higher-risk medical devices tend to be authorized more quickly in the EU than in the United States, where clinical trials are required – but also that patients in Europe may thereby be exposed to medical devices with potentially adverse consequences that are not brought to light by the more limited assessment required.[17] Doubts have also been expressed about the role of NBs in the regulatory process; as private companies whose income derives from the fees that they charge manufacturers, NBs face a contradictory set of objectives, balancing the need to fulfil their obligations with the need also to continue to receive approvals business from manufacturers. There is also a serious lack of data about how effective the controls are in practice, with a lack of public access to data about product licensing or adverse events.[18]

In November 2018 a global investigation known as the "Implant files" revealed the harm caused by medical devices that had been poorly tested in Europe.[19] One significant scandal concerns defective breast implants, known as PIP implants. Manufactured by a French company and marketed in 65 countries around the world, they were available for over a decade with official authorization despite multiple warnings from physicians and despite the fact that the Food and Drug Administration (FDA) had banned these implants from the US market as early as 2000. In total, more than 400 000 women in 65 countries received these implants. On 30 March 2010 the then French Health Products Security Agency (AFSSAPS) announced the recall of PIP implants due to their unusually high rupture rates, combined with the (re)discovery that the manufacturers had been deliberately using unapproved industrial silicone since 2001 in order to save

15 Medtech Europe (2019). Industry Perspective on the Implementation Status of the MDR/IVDR. Available at: https://www.medtecheurope.org/wp-content/uploads/2019/06/2019_MTE_MedTechEurope-IVDR-MDR-Implementation-Status-07-June-2019.pdf.

16 Chai JY (2000). Medical device regulation in the United States and the European Union: a comparative study. *Food and Drug Law Journal*, 55:57.

17 Kramer DB, Xu S, Kesselheim AS (2012). Regulation of medical devices in the United States and European Union. *New England Journal of Medicine*, 366(9):848–55.

18 Kramer DB, Xu S, Kesselheim AS (2012). How does medical device regulation perform in the United States and the European Union? A systematic review. *PLoS Medicine*, 9(7):e1001276.

19 https://www.icij.org/investigations/implant-files/.

money. As ever, crises have a way of driving change, and the Commission has proposed some strengthening of the oversight for medical devices, in particular following serious problems involving these faulty breast implants, vaginal mesh and some hip replacements.[20]

In 2017 the EU passed two new laws intended to address the deficiencies in medical devices regulation.[21] They are intended to be fully effective in 2020 and 2022, replacing the three previous directives on medical devices. The new regulations address some of the weaknesses of the EU regulatory system. First, they seek to increase the transparency of the system through the collation of key supply chain data. The 2017 regulations therefore expand the EU's existing centralized database (EUDAMED) to collect new data on vigilance and post-market surveillance in a form that is supposed to be interoperable with centrally held clinical trials data on pharmaceuticals.[22] Second, the directives also require the creation of a central register of supply chain operators and NBs, as well as the centralization of serious incident reports. Regarding patients, implant recipients will now get "implant cards" describing the type of implants they received. Third, the EU Commission can now investigate when an NB does not seem to be fulfilling its function properly. At the national level, health agencies can conduct unannounced visits and NBs must submit documentation upon request. Finally, national agencies can control an NB's assessment of a manufacturer's documentation before the device is placed on the market.

Although these reforms represent significant improvements to the previous regulatory framework, some components might not be implemented and some key issues are left unaddressed. Industry representatives have raised strong concerns that the timetable for adapting to the new regulations is too tight. As of July 2019, of the approximately 60 NBs in the EU only two had been approved for NB status under the new regulations. Concerns have also been raised about whether or not the EU will deliver on the full promise of EUDAMED due to technical difficulties as well as predictable political difficulties.[23] Failing to approve enough NBs would result in significant consequences for patient access to medical devices across the EU, while a subpar EUDAMED would significantly weaken the impact of the directive on patient safety.

---

20 European Commission (2012). *Communication to the European Parliament, the Council, the European Economic and Social Committee and the Committee of the Regions: safe, effective and innovative medical devices and in vitro diagnostic medical devices for the benefit of patients, consumers and healthcare professionals (COM(2012)540 final)*. Luxembourg: Publications Office of the European Union.

21 Regulation 2017/745 on medical devices (EU IVDR) and Regulation 2017/746 on in vitro diagnostic medical devices (EU IVDR).

22 McHale JV (2018). Health law, Brexit and medical devices: a question of legal regulation and patient safety. *Medical Law International*, 18(2–3):195–215.

23 Medtech Europe (2019). Industry Perspective on the Implementation Status of the MDR/IVDR. Available at: https://www.medtecheurope.org/wp-content/uploads/2019/06/2019_MTE_MedTechEurope-IVDR-MDR-Implementation-Status-07-June-2019.pdf.

Vitally, under the new directives NBs and supply chain operators remain almost entirely responsible for pre-market control. The pre-2017 frameworks remain, in that respect, largely intact, despite the fact that states lack the capacity to effectively control the actions of NBs. Finally, although the EU Commission originally proposed a more centralized system analogous to that embodied by the EMA or the FDA, private actors and NBs lobbied against it.[24] Taken together, both regulations maintain – and only marginally improve – a dangerous situation, which resulted in the past in poor health outcomes for patients receiving defective implants.

4.1.3 Pharmacy

Pharmacies and pharmacists receive much less attention in European policy debates than pharmaceuticals, but it is worth noting the complexity and importance of the field (independent of the issue of drug pricing, and parallel trade which we do not cover[25]). "Pharmacy" means many different things in different countries, and there are often strict rules regarding their locations, hours, ownership and staffing. There has been a long series of challenges to these regulations as contraventions of the freedom to provide services, e.g. from firms that wanted to sell online prescriptions across the EU. The Court, so often open to that kind of deregulatory challenge to apparently discriminatory national policies, has been much less open to them in the case of pharmacy.[26]

4.2 People

A commitment to the mobility of people has been a preoccupation of the EU for as long as there has been an EU: at its inception, Italy was concerned to ensure that its citizens could work in the prosperous coal fields of Belgium and West Germany, and fought for strong free movement provisions that would allow them to do so.[27] In health, today, there are three major issues in the free movement of people. The first is the biggest: the movement and regulation of the healthcare

---

24 Hervey TK, McHale JV (2015). *European Union Law: Themes and Implications*. Cambridge: Cambridge University Press.

25 For a starting point in the public health politics of drug pricing, see Hancher L (2010). "The EU pharmaceuticals market: parameters and pathways", in Mossialos E et al. (eds.). *Health Systems Governance in Europe*. Cambridge: Cambridge University Press, pp. 635–82; Jarman H, McKee M, Hervey TK (2018). Health, transatlantic trade, and President Trump's populism: what American Patients First has to do with Brexit and the NHS. *Lancet*, 392:447–50. For a valuable political analysis that has not dated much, *see* Permanand G (2006). *EU pharmaceutical regulation: the politics of policy-making*. Manchester: Manchester University Press; and Permanand G, Mossialos E (2005). Constitutional asymmetry and pharmaceutical policy-making in the European Union. *Journal of European Public Policy*, 12(4):687–709.

26 For a relatively critical but thorough and lucid analysis of the pharmacy cases to 2011, *see* Hancher L, Sauter W (2012). *EU competition and internal market law in the health care sector*. Oxford: Oxford University Press.

27 Maas W (2007). *Creating European Citizens*. Lanham, MD: Rowman & Littlefield.

workforce within Europe. The second is the movement of patients under social security law, the long-established mechanism for patient mobility that includes the EHIC card. The third deals with migration in and out of the EU itself. In health and in general the movements of the workforce, of consumers and of third country nationals (non-EU citizens) are very different issues.

4.2.1   Health workforce

With 18.6 million workers in 2018, amounting to 8.5% of the total EU workforce, the health workforce is the largest segment of the European labour market.[28] Although the health workforce has grown over the last two decades, this growth was more significant for medical doctors and nurses in the "older" EU Member States. The demand for healthcare professionals in Europe will increase significantly in the next decade as the European population ages and as the number of patients with chronic conditions grows. Such demographic changes will impact the European healthcare workforce in several ways. The growing number of elderly patients with chronic pathologies will require new models of healthcare delivery, which involves expanding physician training. It is also likely to exacerbate the shortage of healthcare professionals that most EU Member States are already facing today. Such shortages are fuelled by factors such as difficulties in recruiting and retaining healthcare professionals, an increasing turnover in the health professions and a growing desire for a better work–life balance that can be difficult to achieve with a medical career.

The 2011 EU research project on Health Professionals Mobility and Health System (PROMeTHEUS) showed that for 17 European countries – including Denmark, Finland, France, Germany and Romania – there was a chronic undersupply of health professionals in rural and sparsely populated areas, and an oversupply of doctors in urban areas, most notably in Germany. The study also showed an oversupply of nurses in Belgium. The PROMeTHEUS study also focused on healthcare professionals' intra-European mobility and concluded that there were significant differences in cross-border movements, with an east-west asymmetry for doctors, nurses and dentists. Western and northern EU countries both experience migration of their healthcare professionals and receive professionals from other countries, while other EU Member States mostly see their clinical workforce shrink due to the departure of their physicians.

In this context, intra-EU health workforce mobility increased over the last two decades in order to address local shortages and as an expression of multiple and sometimes contradictory professional needs at individual and national levels.

---

28 Wismar M et al. (2018). Developments in Europe's Health Workforce: addressing the conundrums. *Eurohealth*, 24(2):38–42. Available at: http://www.euro.who.int/__data/assets/pdf_file/0009/381087/eurohealth-vol24-no2-2018-eng.pdf?ua=1.

The intensification of healthcare professionals' mobility therefore "happened in a context of growing clinical shortage, geographical mis-distribution of skills and staff, as well as of demand for new clinical competences".[29] However, variations in curricula development and acquired knowledge and skills remain. In 2012 the European Commission released an "Action Plan for the EU Health Workforce" in order to propose concrete actions in the following areas: forecasting workforce needs and improving workforce planning methodologies, anticipating future skills needs in the health professions, and sharing good practice on effective recruitment and retention strategies for health professionals.[30]

The Action Plan for the EU Health Workforce was followed by a Joint Action on Workforce Planning and Forecasting (2013–2016), which aimed to advance the issue of healthcare professionals' intra-Europe mobility. Finally, building on the work of the Joint Action for the health workforce, SEPEN – Support for the health workforce planning and forecasting expert network (2017–2018) – was established to develop expert networking to structure and exchange knowledge, map out national health workforce policies in EU countries, foster the exchange of knowledge and good practices on health workforce through European workshops, and provide support to EU countries on national implementation of health workforce planning.

Finally, recent revisions to the European legal framework on professional qualifications also helped support these workforce flows. Harmonizing higher education systems has been a priority for the European Union over the last twenty years. The Bologna process was initiated in the early 2000s to harmonize European higher educational systems. European institutions funded various programmes to stimulate cross-national research and student exchange programmes. These initiatives, however, did not specifically target medical education.[31] Healthcare qualifications may therefore still vary significantly between countries. A few notable exceptions to this observation include the 2005 Professional Qualification Directive,[32] which established the rules for temporary mobility and a system of recognition of qualifications for "professions with harmonized minimum training conditions (i.e. nurses, midwives, doctors (general practitioners

---

29 Wismar M et al. (eds.) (2011). Health professional mobility and health systems. Evidence from 17 European countries. Observatory Study Series No. 23. Copenhagen: WHO Regional office for Europe, on behalf of the European Observatory on Health Systems and Policies. Available at: http://www.euro.who.int/__data/assets/pdf_file/0017/152324/e95812.pdf.

30 European Commission (2012). Commission staff working document on an Action Plan for the EU Health Workforce accompanying the document Communication from the Commission to the European Parliament, the Council, the European Economic and Social Committee, and the Committee of the Regions, towards a Job-rich recovery.

31 Greer SL, Kuhlmann E (2019). "Health and Education Policy: Labour Markets, Qualifications, and the Struggle over Standards", in St John SK & Murphy M (eds.). *Education and Public Policy in the European Union*. London: Palgrave Macmillan, pp. 67–88.

32 Directive 2005/36/EC.

and specialists), dental practitioners, pharmacists, architects and veterinary surgeons". Other healthcare workers, including physiotherapists, do not enjoy automatic recognition.[33]

4.2.2 Social security coordination and the European Health Insurance Card

Since the EU has always partly been about encouraging labour mobility within its borders, it should be no surprise that some of its oldest legislation is about social security coordination. Social security coordination refers to the body of law implemented by Member States which ensures that people can cross borders to work and live, temporarily or permanently, without losing access to social security benefits. It is separate from the issue of "posted workers", which refers to arrangements for people who are employed by a firm in one Member State and sent to work in another. It does not mean that there is a European system of social security, any more than there is a European health system.

These provisions mean that if an individual moves to another country for a job, the social security rights that have been built up (including rights to healthcare) move with the person; similarly, if an individual temporarily travels to another EU country for a purpose such as work, study or holiday and falls ill, he or she is covered and will be treated by that country's health system.[34] However, if someone wishes to go abroad for the purpose of healthcare itself, then these provisions are highly restrictive; prior authorization is required from the domestic authorities, which is very rarely given (not surprisingly, as they have to pay the cost of such healthcare, and generally prefer to provide healthcare domestically). Reflecting these provisions, the volume of patients travelling to other countries in order to receive healthcare within the EU has historically been marginal.

Social security coordination has four principles overall, as stated by DG EMPL:[35]

1. You are covered by the legislation of one country at a time so you only pay contributions in one country. The decision on which country's legislation applies to you will be made by the social security institutions. You cannot choose.

---

33 Greer SL, Kuhlmann E (2019). "Health and Education Policy: Labour Markets, Qualifications, and the Struggle over Standards", in St John SK & Murphy M (eds.). *Education and Public Policy in the European Union*. London: Palgrave Macmillan, pp. 67–88.

34 *See* European Commission (2014). *European Health Insurance Card*. Brussels: European Commission. Available at: http://ec.europa.eu/social/main.jsp?langId=en&catId=559, accessed 14 July 2014.

35 https://ec.europa.eu/social/main.jsp?catId=849.

2. You have the same rights and obligations as the nationals of the country where you are covered. This is known as the principle of equal treatment or nondiscrimination.

3. When you claim a benefit, your previous periods of insurance, work or residence in other countries are taken into account if necessary.

4. If you are entitled to a cash benefit from one country, you may generally receive it even if you are living in a different country. This is known as the principle of exportability.

Because health was long considered as part of the social security system in many Member States, it was not surprising that the core mechanism for handling cross-border healthcare was located in social security coordination. It produces the core, visible, benefit of the European Health Insurance Card (EHIC). There is substantial legal and policy literature on the health policy dimensions of social security coordination.[36] An EHIC is the tangible and portable manifestation of two European rights that the (limited) data on it helps to implement.

The first right is to emergency care on the same terms as citizens when travelling abroad for a short term (around three months or less). Thus, if citizens of a Member State must pay a co-payment for treatment, so must people using an EHIC. The second right is to care in another Member State on the same terms as citizens if the home system has pre-authorized the care.

Member States then settle accounts with each other for EHIC treatment given to each other's citizens. In some cases, as with British and German citizens in Spain, this amounts to both a bargain for the home Member States, since Spanish healthcare costs less, and an economic growth strategy for the sunny parts of Spain where they congregate. It is administered by DG Employment, Social Affairs and Inclusion. The internal politics of how Member States administer EHIC charges and reimbursement are not always straightforward and the EU is sometimes unfairly blamed for distortions created within systems by Member State administrative decisions (e.g. slow reimbursement to providers or underpayments).

The law of social security coordination is made by unanimity in the Council – one of the few areas of EU internal law where this stands. That shows how concerned Member States are to maintain their autonomy, and how easy it is to cause problems with these intricate systems. After a long period of legislative stability under Regulation 1408/71, the EU passed a new pair of regulations in 2010

---

36 Palm W, Glinos IA (2010). "Enabling patient mobility in the EU: between free movement and coordination", in Mossialos E et al. (eds.). *Health Systems Governance in Europe*. Cambridge: Cambridge University Press, pp. 509–61; Hervey TK, McHale JV (2015). *European Union health law*. Cambridge: Cambridge University Press.

that promised "modernized coordination".[37] Modernized coordination is more modern in both technical and social policy terms. In technical terms, it improved on the technology for data transfer that was available in 1971, launching an electronic system for the transfer of social security information between Member States. In social policy terms, it moved social security coordination and rights to social security away from the traditional labour market-based male-breadwinner model by expanding rights to include parental and other leave, and expanding the covered population to include people who were not working (e.g. young, retired or simply not working). A model built around single male guest workers was modernized for the twenty-first-century European economy.

The 2016 Commission Work Package responded to pressure from, in particular, the UK to reduce the benefits available to EU citizens in other countries with a further legislative proposal.[38] It reflected a British political reaction to the large inflow of EU Member State citizens in 2004 and a perception, often exaggerated by the UK media, that immigrants from the rest of the EU were attracted by the UK benefit system and were exploiting it. In the run-up to the Brexit referendum, when the EU was trying to adopt policies that would respond to British preferences, the solution was a proposal for a new Regulation focused on fighting fraud, by enabling better information exchange (by establishing a "further permissive legal basis"[39]), and on tying the location of work more closely to the location in which benefits were paid. The UK was the principal EU Member State in which intra-EU immigration, or the perception of unfair advantages to immigrants from other EU Member States, was a difficult political issue. This was in large part because the UK and Sweden were the only Member States that opened their labour markets to citizens of the CEE accession states in 2004, and therefore saw the largest number of arrivals. Predictably, some other Member States were happy to let the UK draw fire for pressing a restrictionist case they supported. While those tensions around intra-EU migration were present in other Member States, it is unlikely that this issue will retain such prominence

---

37 Regulation (EC) No. 883/2004 of the European Parliament and of the Council of 29 April 2004 on the Coordination of social security systems (*Official Journal*, L 166:1); Regulation (EC) No. 987/2009 of the European Parliament and of the Council of 16 September 2009 laying down the procedure for implementing Regulation (EC) No. 883/2004 on the coordination of social security systems (*Official Journal*, L 284:1).

38 2016/0397 (COD) Proposal for a Regulation of the European Parliament and of the Council amending Regulation (EC) No. 883/2004 on the coordination of social security systems and regulation (EC) No. 987/2009 laying down the procedure for implementing Regulation (EC) No. 883/2004.

39 Regulation of the European Parliament and of the Council amending Regulation (EC) No. 883/2004 on the coordination of social security systems and Regulation (EC) No. 987/2009 laying down the procedure for implementing Regulation (EC) No. 883/2004.

after Brexit.[40] The health effect of the change should lie in two areas: in limiting the number of people in certain categories (e.g. short-term residence) who can claim social security benefits, and in incorporating long-term care into social security coordination.

One point worth underlining in the discussion of social security health mobility is that it is *far more important to patients and health systems than patient mobility under internal market law*. The integrating dynamics of the EU mean that while internal market law, discussed in chapter 4, led to the integration of healthcare as a service subject to EU law, the actual provision of healthcare across borders was a problem that was largely solved in 1971. The legal and political drama that began with the *Kohll* and *Decker* decisions, and which provisionally ended with the Directive on patient rights in cross-border mobility, was about whether healthcare was a service under normal EU law. It was not about the patients. It was never about the patients.[41] It was about who would make health law in Europe, and to what end.

4.2.3 Migrants and health

In recent years a significant number of refugees and other migrants have sought asylum or the opportunity to live and work in the EU. The arrival of particularly large numbers of people at EU borders in 2015–2016, in particular, triggered talk of a migration "crisis".[42] There were some very disparate political responses within different EU Member States, ranging from Germany's welcome to the deployment of armed police by some other Member States. Efforts to allocate refugees across Member States proved politically contentious, as did support for border guards or humanitarian relief workers in states such as Italy and Greece where most migrants first arrived.

While most of these migrants were young and healthy, they had special health needs related to their specific situation, including physical exhaustion, mental stress or unhealthy living conditions that needed to be addressed. Their alleged risk of contracting or spreading communicable diseases, it was felt, required a response. Even if this in the first place was the responsibility of reception

---

40 Maas, W. European Citizenship and Free Movement After Brexit. In SL Greer and J Laible, eds. *The European Union After Brexit*. Manchester: Manchester University Press, 2020. Including because the Court has, in response to the direction of politics, become less expansive in its interpretation of free movement rights including to benefits. Blauberger M et al. (2018). ECJ judges read the morning papers. Explaining the turnaround of European citizenship jurisprudence. *Journal of European Public Policy*, 25(10):1422–41.

41 Greer SL (2008). *Power struggle: the politics and policy consequences of patient mobility in Europe*. Observatoire social européen; Greer SL (2013). Avoiding another directive: the unstable politics of European Union cross-border health care law. *Health Economics, Policy and Law*, 8(4):415–21.

42 It is worth noting that, compared to either the numbers of migrants in states in the European neighbourhood today, or to the numbers of migrants at various times in twentieth-century European history, the numbers of migrants are not large.

countries, the visibility and geographic localization of the arrivals suggested EU action, especially to support those Member States receiving a high number of migrants. In 2016 around €7.5 million was provided to improve healthcare for migrants and training of health professionals. Together with the International Organization for Migration (IOM), the Commission also created a Personal Health Record (with accompanying handbook) to ensure continuity of care for migrants moving around from one Member State to another. As discussed in section 3.7.1, the EU also gave significant aid to countries on its borders, especially Turkey, to host migrants who would otherwise have been able to continue on to EU borders.

4.3   Services

The freedom to provide services across borders in the EU is an important legal principle even if its actual importance in the lives of Europeans differs sharply from sector to sector. In the case of health, the amount of cross-border services that have been delivered is rarely important (with the partial exception of pharmacy, *see* section 4.1.3), but it was as a service across borders that the Court first brought healthcare under EU law in the 1998 *Kohll* and *Decker* rulings, and it is on the freedom to provide services that the key (only) legislation on healthcare systems rests.

4.3.1   Cross-border healthcare and patient mobility

The central issue for health in terms of services is cross-border healthcare. This has been historically very limited within the EU. As discussed in section 4.2.2, there are long-standing provisions on coordination of social security designed to ensure the free movement of workers (social security in EU terms is taken to include healthcare).[43]

The EU law on cross-border care changed fundamentally in 1998, however. Two Luxembourg citizens, Kohll and Decker, argued that they should be able to exercise their right to healthcare in other EU countries and that preventing them from doing so was a barrier to the internal market;[44] the European Court of Justice agreed. This was easier to argue in the case of an insurance-based system such as that in Luxembourg, in which citizens pay for their healthcare initially and are then reimbursed; why should they not be able to purchase their healthcare from a provider just across the border if it does not cost any more? It was less obvious in public provision systems such as the national health service

---

43   European Parliament and Council (2004). Regulation (EC) No. 883/2004 of 29 April 2004 on the coordination of social security systems. *Official Journal*, L 166:1.
44   European Court of Justice. Cases C-158/96 *Kohll*, C-120/95 *Decker*.

Table 4.1 *Comparison between cross-border healthcare rules under the Regulation on Coordination of Social Security and the Directive on Patients' Rights in Cross-Border Healthcare*

	Regulation on Coordination of Social Security	Directive on Patients' Rights in Cross-Border Healthcare
Prior authorization	Required for any planned healthcare in another EU Member State; not required for immediately necessary care while in another EU Member State for other reasons	May be required for hospital care (meaning inpatient care) and other cost-intensive treatments, health hazards and unsuitable providers
Tariffs	The State of treatment; the State where the person is covered if this means more than the State of treatment (up to the level of actual cost)	The State where the person is covered (up to the level of actual cost)
Payment method	Publicly funded element settled between national ministries/insurers	Paid by the patient with subsequent reimbursement by the State where they are covered (unless the State makes direct arrangements to pay)
Provider	Only providers affiliated with the State of treatment social security system	All providers who legally provide healthcare in the State of treatment
Travel and accommodation costs	State of coverage covers costs that are inseparable from the treatment if it would cover them domestically	Covered to the same extent as they would be domestically – although by virtue of being travelling abroad and thus different, what this means in practice is unclear

Source: Greer SL, Sokol T (2014). Rules for rights: European law, health care, and social citizenship. *European Law Journal*, 20(1):66–87.

systems of countries such as Spain, Italy and the United Kingdom, but the Court confirmed through a series of cases that the same legal principles applied.

However, the Court only established the basic principles. It remained up to legislators to decide how to implement them. Given the sensitivities in Member States over health systems, this might have been expected to be a lengthy and fraught process, and indeed it was, taking over a decade before the adoption of the Directive on Patients' Rights in Cross-Border Healthcare in 2011.[45] However, like the Court's original rulings, this system coexists with the original regulations on coordination of social security systems, meaning that there are now two EU systems for cross-border healthcare running in parallel, as set out in Table 4.1.

In practice, and despite the controversy over the Court's rulings, the actual numbers of patients seeking care abroad under the directive remains very low,[46] at around 200 000 per year (though slowly rising), which is only around a tenth of

---

45 European Parliament and Council (2011). Directive 2011/24/EU of 9 March 2011 on the application of patients' rights in cross-border healthcare. *Official Journal*, L 88:45.

46 Report from the Commission to the European Parliament and the Council on the operation of Directive 2011/24/EU on the application of patients' rights in cross-border healthcare; COM(2018)651, 21 September 2018.

the number using the Regulation that provides for the European Health Insurance Card, and a vanishingly small proportion of total care provided domestically.

However, the directive has had larger impacts in other ways. One way has been through domestic measures taken in response to the directive that have a potential impact for all patients, whether travelling abroad or not. Elements of the directive aligned better with some national systems than others, and in some systems the requirements of the directive led to significant domestic change.[47] For example, the logic of the directive required some explicit statement of what was and what was not included as part of a patient's healthcare entitlement, which some systems did not have but introduced following the directive. It also created long waiting times in some cases. Similarly, some systems did not have requirements for liability insurance for professionals in case of problems with care. The directive was also neutral about the public or private status of providers in other countries, which led to discussions in several countries about whether there should be some form of access enabled for private providers within the domestic system. How far these provisions have concretely changed the experience of patients in regard to their health systems is not yet clear. However, it does suggest that the directive has had a wider impact on health systems than simply as regards patients seeking care abroad under its provisions.

The other major impact of the directive is through its ancillary provisions on practical cooperation between European health systems. The Commission took the opportunity of the directive to provide a legal mechanism for greater European cooperation between health systems, building on the issues that emerged from the discussions that led up to the directive, including cross-border recognition of prescriptions, health technology assessment and European Reference Networks (discussed below).

Understanding the impact of the directive requires assumptions about just what it was supposed to do. One of the most obvious objectives was to provide legal certainty: to replace case by case jurisprudence with stable legislation. The track record of this strategy as a way to slow judicial integration is imperfect, since legislation often raises the profile of the issue and makes both lawyers and judges more confident.[48] There is still a risk of that in healthcare.[49] Another is to enhance patients' rights – which makes little sense given that we are still discussing people who choose to seek non-emergency treatment abroad, pay out

---

47 Azzopardi-Muscat N et al. (2018). The role of the 2011 patients' rights in cross-border healthcare directive in shaping seven national health systems: looking beyond patient mobility. *Health Policy*, 122(3):279–83. Available at: https://doi.org/10.1016/j.healthpol.2017.12.010.

48 Kelemen RD (2011). *Eurolegalism: The transformation of law and regulation in the European Union.* Cambridge: Harvard University Press.

49 Greer SL (2013). Avoiding another directive: the unstable politics of European Union cross-border health care law. *Health Economics, Policy and Law*, 8(4):415–21.

of pocket and then seek reimbursement. That is a very small and very specific segment of European society.

A third is to try to improve European healthcare policy by adding dimensions of healthcare improvement to the directive. That certainly happened. The Commission took the opportunity of the directive to provide a legal mechanism for greater European cooperation between health systems, building on the issues that emerged from the discussions that led up to the directive, including cross-border recognition of prescriptions, health technology assessment (discussed in more detail above) and European Reference Networks, despite the reticence of some Member States in both cases. These measures are the subject of sections 4.3.2–5.

4.3.2   European Reference Networks

Under the chapter on cooperation in healthcare within Directive 2011/24/EU, a legal basis was established for the creation of European Reference Networks (ERNs). Article 12 lays out the fundamental principles and objectives for these ERNs. The idea is to link existing centres of expertise in various Member States that are specialized in the diagnosis and care of rare, low prevalence and complex diseases. This should help centralize knowledge and expertise, and strengthen medical research and training, as well as facilitate improvements in diagnosis and treatment for patients with a medical condition that requires a pooling of knowledge and concentration of expertise in medical domains where this expertise is rare.

In a Delegated Decision, the Commission further specified the legal criteria and conditions that ERNs and participating healthcare providers must fulfil.[50] Simultaneously, in an implementing Decision, it detailed the criteria for establishing and evaluating ERNs and their members and for facilitating exchange of information and expertise on establishing and evaluating such networks.[51] In this voluntary process a strong role was attributed to the Member States. The Board of Member States is responsible for developing the overall ERN strategy, approving the networks as well as recognizing the participating centres at national level.

Following the first call for proposals in July 2016, 24 thematic ERNs were approved in December 2016, each one focused around a specific disease area such as bone disorders, haematological diseases, childhood cancer and

---

50 Commission Delegated Decision 2014/286/EU of 10 March 2014 setting out criteria and conditions that European Reference Networks and healthcare providers wishing to join a European Reference Network must fulfil. *Official Journal*, L 147:71.

51 Commission Implementing Decision 2014/287/EU of 10 March 2014 setting out criteria for establishing and evaluating European Reference Networks and their Members and for facilitating the exchange of information and expertise on establishing and evaluating such Networks. *Official Journal*, L 147:79.

immunodeficiency. At their inception in March 2017, the networks comprised more than 900 highly specialized healthcare units located in 313 hospitals in 25 Member States (plus Norway).

Each ERN is led by an ERN coordinator. The ERN Coordinators Group meets three times a year. While clinical services provided in the context of the ERNs are not funded, the various EU funding programmes (Health Programme, Connecting Europe Facility and Horizon 2020) are financially supporting the coordination and management of the ERNs as well as specific functions or projects (e.g. grants for registries or clinical research). In addition, the Commission provides in-kind support with the set-up of a web-based Collaborative Platform (ECP) to stimulate and facilitate collaboration between ERN members, and the establishment of a clinical patient management system (CPMS), which is an IT platform for ERN members to share clinical data on specific patients and organize virtual consultations.

Among the challenges for the ERNs in the coming years are their integration into national health systems and alignment with national strategies on rare diseases, as well as their further enlargement to other providers, including affiliated partners and clinical areas. A recent opinion report by the Expert Panel on Effective Ways of Investing in Health (EXPH) advised against further expanding the ERNs to other areas of healthcare before fully evaluating their costs and benefits.[52] A first evaluation of the ERN initiative is announced for 2021.

4.3.3   The information society and e-health

The concept of e-health can be defined as "the application of information and communications technologies (ICT) across the whole range of functions that affect health".[53] Increasingly, this concept is being broadened to talk about 'digitalization', which expands the concept of e-health to also incorporate the use of data and related systems, such as personal data (e.g. genomic data) or data to support better health and care (e.g. through the use of algorithms or artificial intelligence). Health systems are a sector with enormous potential for improving quality and productivity through application of these technologies, and given the sheer size of health systems in Europe, such improvements would have a

---

52   Expert Panel on Effective Ways of Investing in Health (EXPH), Opinion on the Application of the ERN model in European cross-border healthcare cooperation outside the rare diseases area. European Union, 2018.

53   European Parliament and Council (2011). Directive 2011/24/EU on the application of patients' rights in cross-border healthcare. *Official Journal*, L 88:45; BEUC (2011). *E-Health Action Plan 2012–2020 public consultation*. Brussels: BEUC. Available at: http://www.beuc.org/publications/2011-00398-01-e. pdf, accessed 3 July 2014; Iakovidis I, Purcarea O (2008). "E-Health in Europe: from vision to reality", in Blobel B, Pharow M & Nerich M (eds.). *EHealth: combining health telematics, telemedicine, biomedical engineering and bioinformatics to the edge*. Amsterdam: IOS Press, pp. 163–8.

> **Box 4.2** *General Data Protection Regulation (GDPR)*
>
> A central challenge for the digitalization agenda concerns different and broader uses of personal data. With the rise of information and communication technologies, the use of data about people has become both more visible and more contentious. European legislation on data protection[a] was intended to provide an enabling framework for the movement and use of data, but in practice uncertainty about what is allowed and different interpretations in different countries have meant that legal and political tensions around use of data remain.[b] If the potential of digitalization in health is to be realized, a clear Europe-wide legal framework that commands general public support is required, but this challenge is still far from being met.
>
> ---
>
> [a] Regulation (EU) 2016/679 of the European Parliament and of the Council of 27 April 2016 on the protection of natural persons with regard to the processing of personal data and on the free movement of such data, and repealing Directive 95/46/EC (General Data Protection Regulation). *Official Journal*, L119:1.
>
> [b] Fahy N, Williams G (2019). Building and maintaining public trust to support the secondary use of personal health data. *Eurohealth* 26(2) pp. 7-10.

major impact on the European economy as a whole.[54] The textbook example of the potential for EU standards to generate a market that can drive innovation is the Global System for Mobile Communication (which provides standards for mobile phones) where by establishing a single standard the EU collectively developed a much more advanced mobile phone sector than the other major market at the time, the United States.[55] The equivalent for healthcare is the concept of "interoperability": the idea that individual e-health systems may be different but can still exchange information in a way that can be understood by both.[56] This is straightforward in principle but extremely difficult to make work in practice, and depends on a range of additional elements such as reliable means of identifying individual patients and exchanging highly sensitive data securely.

The Directive on Patients' Rights in Cross-Border Healthcare provides a legal basis for establishing a network on e-health in order to address such practical issues, focusing in particular on cross-border aspects (such as summary records for cross-border care, identification and secure sharing of information), as well as the vital strategic issue of methods for using e-health to enable use of medical information for public health and research – potentially an answer to address the delays that currently plague health data. The European Commission also finances a wide range of projects developing and piloting e-health technologies and applications, for example in support of the European Innovation Partnership

---

54 European Commission (2012). *EHealth Action Plan 2012–2020: innovative healthcare for the 21st century (COM(2012) 736)*. Luxembourg: Publications Office of the European Union.

55 Pelkmans J (2001). The GSM standard: explaining a success story. *Journal of European Public Policy*, 8(3):432–53.

56 *See* Commission Recommendation of 2 July 2008 on cross-border interoperability of electronic health record systems (2008/594/EC). *Official Journal*, L 190:37.

on Active and Healthy Ageing.[57] E-health is presented as a way to address the shortage of health professionals in the European Union, to ensure better care of ageing populations and chronic diseased putting pressure on health budget, as well as to remedy unequal quality and access to healthcare services in Europe.

Reflecting the greater shift towards digitalization, in April 2018 the Commission released a Communication on enabling the digital transformation on health and care in the Digital Single Market,[58] in which it set out its intention to take action in three areas: "citizen's secure access to and sharing of health data across borders; better data to advance research, disease prevention and personalized health and care; digital tools for citizen empowerment and person-centred care".

4.3.4 European prescriptions and the eHealth Digital Service Infrastructure (eHDSI)

Although planned cross-border healthcare is relatively rare, a much more frequent issue is people travelling abroad who for some reason need to have a prescription dispensed – perhaps because they have a chronic condition that requires frequent medication. Yet despite the strongly harmonized European system for licensing pharmaceuticals, such recognition of prescriptions has been historically tricky as it raises a host of practical issues, such as prescriptions written in other languages, or how a pharmacist can be sure of the validity of the prescription or the authority of the doctor to issue it.

This was another issue where the Commission took the opportunity of the Directive on Patients' Rights in Cross-Border Healthcare to make provision for improving European cooperation, through putting in place measures to address such practical database issues (such as by stipulating information to be included on prescriptions that would allow a pharmacist to identify doctors and if necessary contact them).[59]

Directive 2011/24 aims to ensure continuity of care for EU citizens across borders. The Directive allows Member States to exchange health data in a secure and interoperable way. As a result, several services are currently being introduced in all Member States. First, an *ePrescription* and an *e-Dispensation* allow any EU citizen to retrieve his or her medicines from a pharmacy located in another Member State.

---

57 *See* European Commission (2014). *Digital agenda for Europe: ehealth and ageing.* Brussels: European Commission. Available at: http://ec.europa.eu/digital-agenda/en/life-and-work/ehealth-and-ageing, accessed 14 July 2014.

58 European Commission (2018). Communication from the Commission to the European Parliament, the Council, the European Economic and Social Committee and the Committee of the Regions on enabling the digital transformation of health and care in the Digital Single Market; empowering citizens and building a healthier society. Brussels, European Commission, 25 April 2018.

59 European Commission (2012). Commission implementing Directive 2012/52/EU. *Official Journal*, L 356:68.

This is made possible through the electronic transfer of the prescription from the country of residence to the country of travel. Second, *Patient Summaries* provide background information on important medical aspects, including allergies, current medication, previous illness, surgeries, etc. This information is digitally accessible in the event of a medical (emergency) visit in another country. The Commission will present, in the second semester of 2019, a Recommendation on the European Electronic Health Record Exchange Format. Both services were implemented through the *eHealth Digital Service Infrastructure*, which connects the eHealth national services, allowing them to exchange health data. Such infrastructure is funded by the Commission's Connecting Europe Facility.

Since 21 January 2019, for instance, Finnish patients are able to go to any pharmacy in Estonia and retrieve medicines prescribed electronically by their doctor in Finland.[60] The initiative applies to all *ePrescriptions* prescribed in Finland and to the Estonian pharmacies that have signed the agreement. Patients do not have to provide a written prescription; *ePrescriptions* are visible electronically to participating pharmacists in the receiving country via the new *eHealth Digital Service Infrastructure*. As of January 2019, 22 Member States are part of the *eHealth Digital Service Infrastructure* and are expected to exchange *ePrescriptions* and *Patient Summaries* by the end of 2021. In 2018 the Court of Auditors was very critical of the management of this project, which drew on funds from a variety of EU sources;[61] the information exchange between Finland and Estonia was both years late and far more limited than originally planned and hardly EU-wide.

4.3.5   Patient safety and quality

Patient safety is defined as the absence of preventable harm to a patient during the healthcare process. It might seem to be moving a long way from single internal market law and patient mobility, but it is within the framework of patient mobility that the EU has developed a role in patient safety. If there is to be any kind of European market in publicly financed health services, then as with anything else the logic of the European regulatory state demands that it have enough regulation and transparency to be safe even if the number of people using the market is tiny.

Treaty base aside, there is certainly scope for work on the topic. It is estimated that 8–12% of patients admitted to a hospital in the European Union suffer from

60 European Commission. Press Release: "First EU citizens using ePrescriptions in other EU country". Brussels. 21 January 2019.
61 European Court of Auditors Special Report #7 (2019). EU actions for cross-border healthcare: significant ambitions but improved management required.

adverse effects while receiving healthcare, such as healthcare-associated infections, errors in diagnosis, and medication-related and surgical errors.[62]

Issues of patient safety do have a cross-border dimension, both for cross-border care and because health care-associated infections are one of the key potential threats to the safety of patients that can potentially cross borders with a patient. The EU's action is broader, although aiming to support improvements in best practice more generally, given the scope for mutual learning in this area, and best practices were distilled down into a Council Recommendation on Patient Safety, adopted in 2009.[63] While a variety of projects can and have been funded from the health and research programmes on the issue of patient safety, it is possible that the most impact will come from improved, transparent and comparable data if the projects are able to deliver. This may also be supported by the Directive on Patients' Rights in Cross-Border Healthcare, which obliges Member States to ensure transparency about quality and safety standards.

The Commission published a first report in 2012, which demonstrated progress in the development of national policies on patient safety and identified areas requiring further action, including the education and training of healthcare workers in patient safety.[64] In a second report published in 2014,[65] the Commission reported that although the 2009 Recommendation raised political awareness at the political level and triggered changes, it did not necessarily promote a patient safety culture at the healthcare setting level.

4.4   Competition, state aids and services of general interest

The EU has long had strong competition (anti-trust) law, with a powerful executive role for the Commission. Seen as a complement to internal market regulation establishing free movement and fostering free competition across borders, competition law is justified by the goal of ensuring fair competition between enterprises. It is aimed at economic agents (undertakings), prohibiting them from behaving in a way that is likely to distort market competition. However, governments can also distort competition by granting exclusive rights to certain operators or by providing them with state aids. This is likely to be

---

62 European Commission (2017). DG Research and Innovation. Patient Safety. 7 April 2017.

63 Council of the European Union (2009). Council recommendation on patient safety, including the prevention and control of healthcare-associated infections. *Official Journal*, C 151:1.

64 European Commission (2012). Report from the Commission to the Council on the basis of Member States' reports on the implementation of the Council Recommendation (2009/C 151/01) on patient safety, including the prevention and control of healthcare-associated infections (COM(2012) 658 final).

65 European Commission (2014). Report from the Commission to the Council on the implementation of Council Recommendation 2009/C 151/01 on patient safety, including the prevention and control of healthcare-associated infections. Brussels. 19 June 2014.

very relevant for the health sector, with a predominance of public funding and the presence of a variety of actors with variable degrees of scale, autonomy and business orientation.[66]

Whereas the rules on competition are specified directly in the TFEU,[67] the question as to whether and how competition rules apply to health systems remains a source of uncertainty.[68] First, it depends upon the qualification of health services as "economic" and of the actors operating within health system as "undertakings". Given the absence of clear definitions of these concepts, this needed to be clarified by the CJEU, in a similar way to that which happened for the free movement of health services.[69] From this jurisprudence, it appears that it is not the legal status but rather the nature of the activity that is determinant.[70] Even non-profit-making institutions are considered undertakings if they are engaged in activities of an economic nature.[71] However, institutions entrusted with the administration of mandatory schemes of social security, which are based on solidarity and serve an exclusively social function, were excluded from the application of EU competition law as the activities they performed were considered non-economic.[72]

Even if competition rules apply in principle, which seems to be likely for the actual provision of healthcare, the specificity and non-commercial motivations of many activities could justify exemptions or derogations. The legal concept that is used here to shield public, state and welfare services from competition and state aids law is "services of general (economic) interest" (SGEI or SGI).[73] The TFEU explicitly refers to this concept for allowing the setting aside of rules if they would obstruct the performance of SGEIs entrusted to an undertaking.[74]

---

66 Hancher L, Sauter W (2012). *EU competition and internal market law in the health care sector*. Oxford, Oxford University Press.

67 TFEU, Chapter 1 of Title VII, Articles 101–9.

68 Mossialos E, Lear J (2012). Balancing economic freedom against social policy principles: EC competition law and national health systems, *Health Policy*, 106:127–37.

69 *See also* Gekiere W, Baeten R, Palm W (2010). "Free movement of services in the EU and health care", in Mossialos E et al. (eds.). *Health systems governance in Europe: the role of EU law and policy*. Cambridge: Cambridge University Press, pp. 461–508.

70 Prosser T (2010). "EU competition law and public services", in Mossialos E et al. (eds.). *Health systems governance in Europe: the role of EU law and policy*. Cambridge: Cambridge University Press, pp. 315–36.

71 European Court of Justice. Cases C-41/90 *Höfner and Elser*, C-475/99 *Ambulanz Glöckner*, C-67/96 *Albany*, C-180/98–C-184/98 *Pavlov*.

72 European Court of Justice. Cases C-159/91 and C-160/91 *Poucet-Pistre, Garcia, Cisal, FENIN, AOK*.

73 Services of General Interest is a problematic topic. Some EU Member State legal traditions, such as in the UK, have no such concept, or if they do have an equivalent, they formulate it quite differently. Others have a well-developed legal or political concept of SGI, as in France and Germany, but in their legal traditions its meanings and impact vary considerably. One of the problems with the concept is that it therefore generates misunderstanding and has trouble gaining political traction either in the abstract or in any specific formulation. *See* Schweitzer H (2011). "Services of general economic interest: European law's impact on the role of markets and of Member States", in Cremona M (ed.). *Market Integration and Public Services in the European Union*. Oxford: Oxford University Press, pp. 11–62.

74 TFEU, Article 106(2).

Later, as public service sectors increasingly became liberalized, the concept was used to define the scope of regulation to protect and preserve the general good principles of universality, continuity, affordability and quality within these new markets. This required a different approach. With the inclusion of a specific article on services of general interest in the Amsterdam Treaty in 1997, the focus shifted away from a mere derogation towards a positive duty for Member States and the EU to promote SGEIs.[75] While a derogation needs to be interpreted strictly and with due respect to proportionality, the new legal base of Article 14 of the TFEU allows for a more proactive and systematic approach, with the EU adopting regulations to further define operational principles and conditions for SGEIs to ensure achieving their mission. Although in a Protocol attached to the TFEU, the concept and role of SGEIs, as well as their underpinning principles and values, are further elaborated, a broader and consistent regulatory framework is still lacking, probably partly because of the diversity of legal traditions that use variations on the concept.[76]

Instead the European Commission has been developing – also based on CJEU jurisprudence – a set of criteria to define SGEIs and the scope for derogation to be granted. In 2004, in its White Paper on Services of General Interest,[77] the Commission announced a specific Communication on Social and Health Services of General Interest, to identify and recognize these and to clarify the framework in which they operate and can be modernized. However, after health services were excluded from the Services Directive,[78] they were also excluded from the scope of this Communication in 2006,[79] the claim being that they would be covered in the upcoming Directive on Patient Rights' in Cross-Border Healthcare. However, while this directive did address the reimbursement of cross-border health services, it did not cover the wider application of internal market rules on the health sector.

---

75 Szyszcak E (2007). "Competition law and services of general economic interest", in ERA Conference on European integration and national social protection systems: towards a new form of internal market. Brussels, 31 May–1 June, 2007.

76 Schweitzer H (2011). "Services of general economic interest: European law's impact on the role of markets and of Member States", in Cremona M (ed.). *Market Integration and Public Services in the European Union*. Oxford: Oxford University Press, pp. 11–62.

77 European Commission (2004). Commission to the European Parliament, the Council, the European Economic and Social Committee and the Committee of the Regions. *White paper on services of general interest (COM/2004/0374 final)*. Luxembourg: Publications Office of the European Union.

78 European Parliament and Council (2006). *Directive 2006/123 on services in the internal market*. Luxembourg: Publications Office of the European Union.

79 European Commission (2006). *Implementing the Lisbon programme: social services of general interest in the European Union (COM(2006) 177final)*. Luxembourg: Publications Office of the European Union. In 2019 DG COMP (Competition) consulted on an evaluation "to check if the rules on health and social services of general economic interest ... meet their objectives under the 2012 services package". *See* https://ec.europa.eu/info/law/better-regulation/initiatives/ares-2019-3777435_en

One particular area that has attracted a lot of attention in the health sector was "state aid". State aids refer to assistance from public bodies to private undertakings, for example subsidies. On the one hand, these can distort competition, which means that much EU law is hostile to them. On the other hand, subsidies to private or non-profit-making undertakings are often an ordinary part of health systems. The potential clash between state aid law and health system practice has caused some concern and led the EU to develop an elaborate framework to monitor and sanction financial discrimination of economic operators. As state aid is an exclusive EU competency, the Commission's decisions here are crucial. Since 2005 the European Commission has further specified the rules for state funding of SGEIs with the so-called Altmark package (referring to the European Court of Justice case concerning Altmark, a German bus company awarded state aid[80]), which is also known as the Monti–Kroes package,[81] updated in 2012 by the Almunia package. Essentially, if public funding merely compensates for the fulfilment of public service obligations, it is not regarded as state aid. Following the CJEU rulings,[82] this is subject to strict criteria: there needs to be an explicit mandate as well as objective and transparent parameters for calculating the compensation, which cannot exceed actual costs.[83] Even if not all of these Altmark criteria are fulfilled, state aids can still be declared compatible (in advance) without the need for prior notification to the Commission. This applies to a range of mostly social services of a local nature, including hospitals and other care organizations.[84] In addition, a special *de minimis* rule applies, allowing local authorities to provide for smaller amounts of public support that does not affect intercountry trade.[85] In this way it might seem as if the effect of competition and state aid rules on the health sector is limited to, for example, competition in the pharmaceutical sector, although some would argue that the legal uncertainty would force them to adopt hiding and distraction strategies and other unusual

---

80 European Court of Justice. Case C-280/00 *Altmark*.

81 European Commission (2005). *Commission Decision of 28 November 2005 on the application of Article 86(2) of the EC Treaty to state aid in the form of public service compensation granted to certain undertakings entrusted with the operation of services of general economic interest (2005/842/EC).* Brussels: European Commission.

82 European Court of Justice. Cases C-280/00 *Altmark*, C-53/00 *Ferring*.

83 European Commission (2012). Communication on the application of the European Union state aid rules to compensation granted for the provision of services of general economic interest. *Official Journal,* C 8:4.

84 European Commission (2012). Decision of 20 December on the application of Article 106(2) of the Treaty on the Functioning of the European Union to state aid in the form of public service compensation granted to certain undertakings entrusted with the operation of services of general economic interest. *Official Journal,* L 7:3.

85 European Commission (2014). Regulation (EC) No. 1407/2013 of 18 December 2013 on the application of Articles 107 and 108 of the Treaty on the Functioning of the European Union to de minimis aid. *Official Journal,* L 352:1–8; *see also* European Commission (2014). *Block exemption regulations.* Brussels: European Commission. Available at: http://ec.europa.eu/competition/state_aid/legislation/block.html, accessed 28 July 2014.

organizational relationships that might not be efficient, transparent, solidaristic or flexible.[86]

4.4.1 Public and private partnerships

The EU position with regard to public and private partnerships (PPPs) emerges from the interaction of two legal facts. One is that the EU has very powerful legal instruments to enforce fair public procurement procedures. The other is that it has comparatively limited powers or responsibilities for commissioning services. The result is that there are two faces of EU PPP policy: the smaller issue of using PPPs in EU-financed projects and the larger issue of determining whether EU legal frameworks are helpful for those who would use PPPs.

The first issue, concerning the use of PPPs in EU-financed projects (principally meaning projects financed by the structural and cohesion funds and research projects), was discussed in a wide-ranging 2009 Commission Memorandum.[87] The Memorandum simultaneously noted the potential usefulness of PPPs (in light of what it saw as vast future obligations for infrastructure investment) and committed the Commission to their use, but stressed the difficulty of untangling the potential legal issues involved. Most of the examples of PPPs that the Communication discussed were actually in the co-financing of research programmes with private firms. It noted that

> "the Commission is aware of difficulties in combining different sets
> of EU and national rules, practices and timetables. The Commission
> therefore intends to review the rules and practices to ensure that PPPs
> are not put at a disadvantage and issue the necessary guidance to assist
> the public authorities in the preparation of projects."

This puts the focus on the bigger issue with PPPs: not whether the EU is using them in its programmes for financing action but rather whether the EU is failing to strike the right balance between its goal of free and equal access to public markets and the practicalities of bidding on PPPs. Use of PPPs was the subject of a Commission Green Paper in 2004,[88] followed by a consultation and

---

86 Hervey TK (2011). "If only it were so simple: public health services and EU law", in Cremona M (ed.). *Market integration and public services in the European Union.* Oxford: Oxford University Press, pp. 179–250. For the situation with regard to the work of competition authorities in the pharmaceutical sector, *see* "Competition Enforcement in the Pharmaceutical Sector (2009-2019): European competition authorities working together for affordable and innovative medicines" COM(2019)17.

87 European Commission (2009). *MEMO/09/509: Commission communication on public private partnerships – frequently asked questions.* Brussels: European Commission. Available at: http://europa.eu/rapid/pressReleasesAction.do?reference=MEMO/09/509&format=HTML&aged=0&language=EN&guiLanguage=en, accessed 14 July 2014.

88 European Parliament, the Council, the European Economic and Social Committee and the Committee of the Regions (2004). *Green paper on public–private partnerships and community law on public contracts and concessions (COM(2004) 327).* Luxembourg: Publications Office of the European Union.

a 2005 Communication.[89] In the Communication, the Commission concluded that further legislation would probably introduce new complexity and that the implementation of public procurement law need not present difficulties to public or private sector participants. In particular, the procedure of "competitive dialogue" offered the possibility of letting potential commissioners and providers have in-depth discussions without violating public procurement law – a potential problem given that standard public procurement law dissuades close interaction between potential vendors and potential buyers. Another particular issue is that of "concessions", where the private sector provides services together with public authorities (e.g. toll roads); the European Parliament has recently adopted new rules on concessions, as well as updated rules on public procurement.[90]

In practice making use of PPPs is risky and requires considerable expertise.[91] This is one of the key issues highlighted by national representatives themselves in the "toolbox" on the use of the structural funds for health (section 5.4).[92] It remains to be seen whether Member States (separately or working together) can build up greater expertise in using PPPs for health investing in the light of increasing pressure on public budgets. There is also the question of how far liabilities built up through PPP projects do or should count as public debt; in the United Kingdom, for example, which has made extensive use of PPPs in sectors including health over recent decades, these additional liabilities have been estimated at £33 billion, and concern has been expressed that financing is being sought through the PPP route even where this does not represent best value for money in order to keep the resulting liabilities from counting as public debt.[93]

---

89 European Parliament, the Council, the European Economic and Social Committee and the Committee of the Regions (2005). *Communication on public–private partnerships and community law on public procurement and concessions (COM(2005) 569)*. Luxembourg, Publications Office of the European Union.

90 *See* European Parliament (2014). *Press release: new EU-procurement rules to ensure better quality and value for money*. Brussels: European Parliament. Available at: http://www.europarl.europa.eu/news/en/news-room/content/20140110IPR32386/html/New-EU-procurement-rules-to-ensure-better-quality-and-value-for-money, accessed 14 July 2014.

91 Lieberherr E, Maarse H, Jeurissen P (2015). "The governance of public–private partnerships", in Greer SL, Wismar M & Figueras J (eds.). *Strengthening health systems governance: Better policies, stronger performance*. Maidenhead: Open University Press; *see also* Expert Panel on Effective Ways of Investing in Health (2014). *Health and economic analysis for an evaluation of the public–private partnerships in health care delivery across Europe*. Brussels: DG Health and Consumer Protection. Available at: http://ec.europa.eu/health/expert_panel/experts/working_groups/index_en.htm, accessed 14 July 2014.

92 General Secretariat of the Council (2013). *Reflection process: towards modern, responsive and sustainable health systems (12981/13 ADD 2)*. Luxembourg: Publications Office of the European Union, *see* section 5.

93 House of Commons Treasury Committee (2012). *Private finance initiative: government, OBR and NAO responses to the seventeenth report from the committee (HC 1725)*. London: The Stationery Office.

4.5 Innovation Union Partnership on active and healthy ageing

One of the seven *flagship initiatives* proposed by the Juncker Commission to take forward the Europe 2020 strategy was the "Innovation Union",[94] the aim of which is to improve the innovativeness of Europe and ensure that research is effectively translated into practice in sectors including health. One of the key issues identified is the challenges brought by demographic ageing – while the increasing lifespan of Europeans is an excellent outcome of improving living standards and health systems, it also presents significant challenges, with increasing costs to health and social care systems alongside a relative reduction in the size of the working-age population that can keep working to pay for these systems.[95] While the relative size of increases in costs to health systems for the coming decades is actually smaller than the average increases in healthcare spending in the past decades of the EU, this is still a substantial shift and presents a major challenge to countries whose public budgets are already under serious pressure. There is a real risk of counterproductive policies that merely redistribute risk and ultimately cost more by being adopted instead of adopting positive-sum ageing policies.[96]

The Commission accordingly took this topic of "health and active ageing" as the focus of its first Innovation Union Partnership[97] proposed as part of the Innovation Union initiative. The aim of this partnership is to bring together stakeholders and experts across the innovation chain from basic research to practical application in order to improve health, improve the sustainability of health systems and create business opportunities for health industries – indeed, the partnership aimed to increase by two the years of healthy life lived throughout Europe by 2020. This bold objective, however, did not have any additional resources provided to help to achieve it. The partnership depended on existing funding streams at European or national level being voluntarily mobilized to support its priorities, and it relied on the power of its vision to convince actors in the area to take forward the issues that it identified as priorities. Quite a number

94 European Commission (2010). European Parliament, Council, European Economic and Social Committee and Committee of the Regions. *Communication: Europe 2020 flagship initiative innovation union (COM(2010)546)*. Brussels, European Commission.

95 European Commission (ECFIN) and the Economic Policy Committee (AWG) (2009). *The 2009 ageing report: economic and budgetary projections for the EU-27 Member States (2008–2060)*. Brussels: European Commission. Available at: http://ec.europa.eu/economy_finance/publications/publication14992_en.pdf, accessed 4 July 2014.

96 Cylus J, Normand C, Figueras J (2019). Will population ageing spell the end of the welfare state? A review of evidence and policy options. Copenhagen: WHO Regional office for Europe, on behalf of the European Observatory on Health Systems and Policies.

97 European Commission (2013). *European innovation partnership on active and healthy ageing*. Brussels: European Commission. Available at: http://ec.europa.eu/research/innovation-union/index_en.cfm?section=active-healthy-ageing&pg=home, accessed 4 July 2014.

of organizations became involved in the partnership.[98] As of the 2016 data (the latest available), healthy life years in the EU had increased by 1.1 for men and 1.3 for women, though some countries lost healthy life years in that period.[99] The impact of the relatively limited EU programme, with its disparate objectives, in that outcome is unclear. It is, however, useful to expand understanding of the ways that healthy and active ageing policies can contribute to the sustainability of budgets, economies and society.

4.6 Health technology assessment

Health technology assessment (HTA) is the activity of assessing the effectiveness of medical procedures and technologies. It normally does this by comparing treatments in light of therapeutic effectiveness, side-effects, administration and impact on the patient's quality of life. In the famous UK case of NICE, the National Institute for Health and Clinical Excellence, it also involves price, determining whether a given intervention at a given price is justified.[100] Most other HTA agencies focus on value for money, comparing the other dimensions of a treatment's effectiveness (e.g. assessing whether a new treatment's method of administration or therapeutic effectiveness is superior to the existing treatments and leaving it to some other part of the health system to decide whether it is included in the basket of covered services and at what price).

While there is no imperative to pursue European HTA action,[101] there is a case for European coordination and resource pooling in the area of HTA: it is often expensive, requires a range of diverse skills and has a high price of entry, there is an endless supply of medical treatments and technologies that could benefit from HTA, and the EU can seek added value by reducing duplication through better coordination of Member State initiatives. It can also thereby overcome the collective action failure we currently see, in which not all Member States invest in HTA,[102] which means the developing international HTA literature

---

98 European Commission (2013). See the Commission's report on achievements and impact: European Innovation Partnership on Active and Healthy Ageing. *Action groups: first year report*. Brussels: European Commission. Available at: http://ec.europa.eu/research/innovation-union/pdf/active-healthy-ageing/achievements_2013.pdf#view=fit&pagemode=none, accessed 4 July 2014.

99 Eurostat data. Available at: https://ec.europa.eu/eurostat/statistics-explained/index.php/Healthy_life_years_statistics#Healthy_life_years_at_birth.

100 Williams I (2013). Institutions, cost-effectiveness analysis and healthcare rationing: the example of healthcare coverage in the English National Health Service. *Policy & Politics*, 41(2):223–39; Williams I (2016). "The governance of coverage in health systems: England's National Institute for Health and Care Excellence (NICE)", in Greer SL, Wismar M & Figueras J (eds.). *Strengthening Health System Governance*, Open University Press, pp. 159–71.

101 Greer SL, Löblová O (2017). European integration in the era of permissive dissensus: Neofunctionalism and agenda-setting in European health technology assessment and communicable disease control. *Comparative European Politics*, 15(3):394–413.

102 Löblová O (2018). When epistemic communities fail: exploring the mechanism of policy influence. *Policy Studies Journal*, 46(1):160–89.

does not reflect their needs and priorities while also putting more of the burden on a smaller number of Member States which are investing primarily for their own reasons. On the other hand, HTA is not an obvious political winner. It has upfront costs, diffuse and uncertain benefits, and can incur instant opposition from industry and providers,[103] which explains why its diffusion is not as rapid or extensive as its promise to rationalize health technology and care might lead one to expect.[104]

The EU has been involved in HTA for almost as long as there has been such a field: the International Journal of Technology Assessment dates to 1985 and the European "Methodology of Economic Appraisal of Health Technology" to 1986.[105] EU-funded programmes have been running almost continuously since the 1990s, building up to today's EUnetHTA, a joint action funded by the Health Programme. It runs until 2020 and brings together organizations interested in HTA from all the Member States. Its activities are diverse, ranging from diffusing assessments to facilitating its members in conducting joint assessments on technologies. It also has a collaboration with EMA and a joint work plan focused on connecting market authorization with HTA. The Directive on Patients' Rights in Cross-Border Healthcare[106] created a Health Technology Assessment Network (HTA Network) of Member States, which has been meeting since 2013 and is in principle supported for scientific purposes by EUnetHTA. It is a "formalistic grouping of officials from Member States' health ministries, rather than a collaboration of HTA experts".[107]

So far we can view this as a classic case of how European integration develops: by gradually creating a European constituency that sees value added, collectively and individually, in pooling their efforts via EU-level mechanisms, in the same way that communicable disease control or medicines regulation was gradually Europeanized. Predictably enough, the next step was a Commission proposal for legislation to institutionalize HTA at the European Union level.[108] The instrument chosen by the Commission surprised some observers: a Regulation that would

103 The United States is a useful cautionary tale: Gray BH, Gusmano MK, Collins SR (2003). AHCPR and the Changing Politics of Health Services Research: Lessons from the falling and rising political fortunes of the nation's leading health services research agency. *Health Affairs*, 22(Suppl 1):W3–283; Sorenson C, Gusmano MK, Oliver A (2014). The politics of comparative effectiveness research: lessons from recent history. *Journal of Health Politics, Policy and Law*, 39(1):139–70.

104 Löblová O (2018). What has health technology assessment ever done for us? *Journal of Health Services Research and Policy*, 23(2):134–6.

105 For a political history, *see* Greer SL, Löblová O (2017). European integration in the era of permissive dissensus: Neofunctionalism and agenda-setting in European health technology assessment and communicable disease control. *Comparative European Politics*, 15(3):394–413.

106 Directive 2011/24/EU on the application of patients' rights in cross-border healthcare.

107 Löblová O (2018). Epistemic communities and experts in health policy-making. *European Journal of Public Health*, 28(suppl 3):7–10.

108 COM(2018) 51 final, 2018/0018 (COD) Proposal for a Regulation of the European Parliament and of the Council on health technology assessment and amending Directive 2011/24/EU. Brussels, 31.1.2018.

create a formal structure of collaboration between Member States overseen by an EU-level committee. There would be "joint clinical assessments", classic HTA work, as well as more forward-looking "joint scientific consultations" on developing technologies and "horizon-scanning" reports on "emerging health technologies". The Commission would be the secretariat for this structure, providing scientific (advice and stakeholder management) as well as administrative support.

The Commission proposal was published in January 2018. By the end of the Juncker Commission it was the only health dossier of consequence still open, despite the support of the 2019 Romanian and Finnish presidencies. The key obstacle was a variety of Member States that objected on grounds including subsidiarity, ranging from the Czech Republic to France. The response of the Romanian and Finnish presidencies was to lead the redrafting of large parts of the proposal, emphasizing its technical nature and non-duplication of Member State efforts. Its fate as of the end of 2019 remains unclear.

4.7 Trade and investment

The EU is a powerful actor in international trade, aiming to represent its Member States with a single voice in trade and investment negotiations and disputes. The EU has exclusive competence in almost all areas to conduct international negotiations on trade deals, although some practical difficulties remain regarding the sometimes blurred dividing line between international trade and "domestic" EU policy areas, including health. The EU's current and future trade and investment commitments remain intimately connected to the ways in which health service providers, medical professionals, patient mobility and products affecting public health – from food, alcohol and tobacco to pharmaceuticals and medical devices – are regulated within the EU. Awareness of the EU's trade policies is therefore vital for health officials within the EU and at Member State level and dialogue between trade and health officials should be promoted.

The EU is party to many different trade and investment agreements that have implications for health policies. Of the multilateral agreements governed by the World Trade Organization, the most significant for health are the General Agreement on Tariffs and Trade, which governs trade in goods; the General Agreement on Trade in Services, which permits members including the EU to make commitments to liberalize their services markets; the trade-related aspects of the Intellectual Property Rights (TRIPS) agreement, which notably affects patents and access to medicines and has been the subject of much dispute; the Agreement on the Application of Sanitary and Phytosanitary Measures, which addresses the application of food safety and animal and plant health standards with a view to identifying protectionist measures; and the Agreement on Technical

Barriers to Trade, which focuses on the identification of regulatory barriers to trade and has been central to a number of tobacco-related trade disputes.

Outside these multilateral negotiations, the EU has concluded many regional and bilateral trade and investment agreements. These agreements tend to mirror the breadth of the existing multilateral agreements and frequently go beyond them in terms of the level of trade liberalization, intellectual property protections or investor protections that they contain.

Trade agreements and institutions present opportunities to govern the trade of goods and services in ways which can affect health. How this plays out in practice depends not just on the framing of health within these institutions and laws, but also on the intent of the actors operating within them. The extent to which the global trading system impacts health depends upon the ways in which political actors use the system and the goals that they pursue – which may or may not be health goals.

To date, the EU has shown considerable reluctance to make liberalizing commitments directly affecting health services under its trade agreements and has striven to balance access to medicines with protecting its pharmaceutical industry in TRIPS-related discussions and debates. This reflects both the unease of Member States regarding EU policies that could destabilize their healthcare systems, and the concerns of the public and public advocacy groups surrounding health access. Under the TFEU, the EU's trade policy became part of the ordinary legislative procedure, granting an expanded role for the European Parliament in trade policy decision-making. Nevertheless, any agreement in health services "where these agreements risk seriously disturbing the national organization of such services and prejudicing the responsibility of Member States to deliver them" requires unanimous approval from Member States.

Public health advocates have strongly criticized what they view as a lack of transparency and attention to public interest issues in recent trade negotiations. In the case of the Anti-Counterfeiting Trade Agreement (ACTA), an intellectual property agreement negotiated among the EU, United States and nine other industrialized states, these concerns were shared by the European Parliament, which voted against the legislation by 478 votes to 39, with 165 MEPs abstaining. This vote reflected "unprecedented direct lobbying by thousands of EU citizens who called on it to reject ACTA, in street demonstrations, e-mails to MEPs and calls to their offices". Similar concerns have been raised by advocacy groups regarding the now defunct Transatlantic Trade and Investment Partnership, particularly in regard to proposals to include an Investor-State Dispute Settlement (ISDS) procedure – a type of redress mechanism that allows firms to initiate

---

Box 4.3   *Trade and Brexit*

Separating the economy of the United Kingdom from the EU's single market is extremely difficult. For decades the UK has contributed to the direction of EU trade policy and formed part of the market for goods, services and investment from other Member States. The deep political divides in the UK, of which Brexit is a symptom, are likely to last a generation and will continue to make it difficult for EU Member States to define their trading relationship with the UK going forward.

Any economic disruption from Brexit comes with health consequences for Europeans as well as for the British, e.g. in terms of lost revenue, employment or income. In the short to medium term, Brexit (particularly under a "No Deal" scenario) is likely to mean disruptions in trade with effects on health, e.g. interruptions to the supply chains for medicines and medical devices. Brexit planning has already caused some distortions in the market in these areas.

In the long term, the UK's departure means that the EU is losing one of the strongest voices in the bloc in favour of free trade and market liberalization. The internal politics of EU trade is likely to change as a result. It is possible that this could actually have a positive impact on health policy, with reduced pressure to liberalize health services through trade negotiations, for example. However, the balance of politics within the EU-27 could still favour populists who oppose both free trade *and* health, potentially jeopardizing any attempts to balance economic growth with promoting high health standards.[a]

---

[a]   Jarman H. European Union Trade Policy in the Wake of the Brexit Vote. 162–176 in Greer SL and Laible J, eds. *The European Union After Brexit.* Manchester University Press, 2020.

---

international commercial arbitration directly against governments in response to policies perceived as unfair, unreasonable or disproportionate.[109]

The EU and its Member States can also be the targets of trade or investment disputes. Firms have used these mechanisms to challenge the regulations in a number of health-related areas, including chemicals, medicines, the environment and tobacco. The willingness of the tobacco industry to utilize these mechanisms against states regulating tobacco product packaging may well have implications for current and future tobacco control legislation within the EU.

---

109 For ISDS and health in general, *see* Jarman H (2014). *The politics of trade and tobacco control.* London: Palgrave Macmillan. For more detail on the EU dimensions, see Jarman H, Koivusalo M (2017). "Trade and health in the European Union", in Hervey TK, Young C & Bishop L (eds.). *Research Handbook on EU Health Law and Policy.* Cheltenham: Edward Elgar Publishing, pp. 429–52. For TTIP in particular, *see* Jarman H (2014). Public health and the Transatlantic Trade and Investment Partnership. *European Journal of Public Health*, 24(2):181.

4.8 Conclusion

The internal market is, over time, the most demonstrably important face of the EU. It undergirds the wide variety of important policies we have discussed here. But to dismiss the EU as a simple market-making machine is a mistake. Rather, note the wide variety of policies that are made that have important health dimensions and are grounded in internal market law. They include a number of policies with potential value for health systems, such as HTA and workforce, as well as policies which help citizens, such as social security mobility, and ones whose positive contribution is largely unclear, such as the European court rulings on patient mobility or the application of state aids law. If we widen the perspective still further, we note that many broader policies affecting health were for a long time made as part of the single market, since setting regulatory floors often involves raising regulatory standards.

For better or for worse, the regulation of the single internal market is at the core of EU powers. That means that internal market principles – freedom of movement and nondiscrimination – are powerful bases for action that courts will support. It means that much of the EU's positive effect on health is through regulations grounded in the internal market. The question for health is: how do we ensure that the second face of EU health policy smiles on valuable health policies and objectives?

Chapter 5

Fiscal governance of health

The EU treaties specify that the organization and finance of healthcare is a Member State competence (Article 168). That means an observer in 2015 might have been surprised to find that France was being instructed to review the *numerus clausus* for health professional education, or Austria to set and hit quantitative targets for moving treatments out of hospital environments.[1] What happened? How can the same EU that is so tightly bound to a supportive role for Member State action in one part of the treaties be authorized to fine France for its medical school admissions policies in another part?

The answer is the third face of European Union health policy: the impact of fiscal governance on health systems and policies. "Fiscal governance" means EU powers to shape the fiscal policies and stances of Member States both directly, in their spending and taxing decisions, and indirectly, in the kinds of economies they shape and the risks they create. Health is, directly, a very expensive item in any EU Member State, and so if the EU is concerned about budgetary rigour, it is going to be concerned about healthcare expenditures. If the EU is concerned about the long-term fiscal and economic viability of its Member States, then healthcare is indirectly important since it is a key way to invest in a healthy and active workforce (often code for "find a viable way to raise the age of pension eligibility"), address territorial and class inequalities, and reduce the costs associated with poor health.

5.1   How "fiscal governance" came to exist and to matter to health

Fiscal governance in the EU is intimately associated with the project of monetary union that created the Euro. Member States have therefore been developing and experimenting with fiscal governance for decades. The template for fiscal governance that they came to apply to health after 2010 was developed over decades by policy-makers whose concerns were far from those of health systems and health policy-makers.

---

1   Greer S, Jarman H, Baeten R (2016). The New Political Economy of Health Care in the European Union: The Impact of Fiscal Governance. *International Journal of Health Services*, 46(2).

Since the end of the Bretton Woods system of controlled exchange rates in 1973, EU Member States have sought to stabilize exchange rates against each other and promote the political project of monetary union. This entailed the first efforts to harmonize Member States' fiscal stances and economies, and therefore the first forms of fiscal governance.[2] The basic problem was expressed in terms of "credible commitment": Member States' ability to make a commitment on taxes and spending that they would hold to and markets would believe. If such commitments were not credible, bond markets would undermine their currencies and debts, as happened to the United Kingdom in September 1992 when it was unable to remain in the European monetary system at the exchange rate it had chosen.

The 1992 Maastricht Treaty, with its commitment to monetary union for all EU Member States except the UK, raised the stakes. The basic problem is simple enough to describe. The EU Member States, or even the contemporary Eurozone Member States, have very dissimilar economies with different structural advantages and problems vis-à-vis each other and the rest of the world. One of the key ways in which different economies manage their divergences is through fluctuating exchange rates. Thus, for example, countries with higher inflation tended to have depreciating currency vis-à-vis countries with lower inflation. In a monetary union, currency fluctuations cannot compensate for differences. Economies have to become more similar: similar debt, deficits, inflation and macroeconomic structures. One way to do this is to develop powerful economic mechanisms of equalization within the currency union, in the same way that individual countries equalize. Such mechanisms can mean equalizing between citizens across their territories: public sector systems such as healthcare, pensions, education and unemployment benefits redistribute within countries from stronger to weaker economies. The EU, as discussed, has no such redistributive role and there is little support for any such role. It can also mean redistribution between governments, as we see in most federations. The structural funds equalize to a limited extent between governments. But while they play such a big part in the politics and economics of some of the poorer Member States, they comprise a far smaller expenditure as a percentage of GDP than would be required to equalize among EU regions and produce real convergence across the EU as a whole.

The solution at Maastricht was an increase in the intensity and importance of fiscal governance.[3] On one hand, accession to the single currency would require that countries hit a number of important targets, including a deficit less than 3% of GDP and total public debt of less than 60% of GDP. Hitting such targets would require a strong and lasting commitment to public sector

2   James H (2012). *Making the European Monetary Union*. Cambridge: Harvard University Press.
3   Dyson K (2014). *States, Debt, and Power: "saints" and "sinners" in European History and Integration*. Oxford: Oxford University Press.

budgetary rigour. On the other hand, in case such a commitment faded, the Eurozone states signed a Stability and Growth Pact (SGP) which enshrined the deficit and debt targets in law and coupled them with a mechanism to identify and punish Member States that transgressed the limits. The SGP included an element of fiscal governance: the Broad Economic Policy Guidelines (BEPG) which reviewed Member State public policies and their effects on their overall fiscal future and SGP compliance.

In the end, when the final list of countries for monetary union was put together, the 3% and 60% targets were loosened so that Member States could be admitted if they were making credible progress towards those targets (otherwise the Eurozone would have had only a few members, none of them big countries). The Euro launched in 2000. Without the pressure to achieve Eurozone membership criteria, Member States would now be disciplined by the SGP and the BEPG and, to an unknown extent, the markets.

The post-2000 fiscal governance system did not fare very well. In 2005 the Commission found that both France and Germany were clearly in violation of the SGP. To little surprise, their leaders persuaded the Council to rewrite the SGP. After 2005 it would reward adoption of policies that, the Council judged, would lead to sustainable fiscal performance (e.g. Germany was in violation partly because of the costs of its Hartz IV employment policy package, which the German government argued was an investment in a more solid German economy).[4] Only one Member State – Ireland – was ever criticized under the BEPG, and it ignored the criticism.[5] These events had little impact on policy or the Eurozone economies at the time, but they sapped credibility from the EU fiscal governance system. It could evidently be rewritten or defied by large and small countries. Eurozone economies continued to benefit from economic growth, currency unification, the free flow of capital and the low borrowing costs of Eurozone Member States.

The economic crisis that began in 2010 was a result of a global economic crisis triggered by misbehaviour and imbalances within the financial sector but it manifested in Europe in the form of a sovereign debt crisis. Essentially, the problem was that some economies had responded to the Euro since 2000 with wage constraint, which meant that they became more competitive and grew, accumulating surpluses vis-à-vis other Eurozone Member States. Others, with less coordinated labour markets, suffered inflation and saw sectors such as tourism or the public sector (including healthcare) grow at the expense of sectors such as

---

4   Schelkle, W (2009). The Contentious Creation of the Regulatory State in Fiscal Surveillance. *West European Politics*, 32:829–46.
5   Deroose S, Hodson D, Kuhlmann J (2008). The Broad Economic Policy Guidelines: Before and After the Re-Launch of the Lisbon Strategy. *JCMS: Journal of Common Market Studies*, 46:827–48.

manufacturing. The result was growing imbalances: higher and higher surpluses in northern creditor countries, which exported their surplus funds to peripheral countries in various forms including bank loans, purchase of government debt, real estate investment and tourism. When the financial crisis halted economic growth and reduced investment across borders, the countries dependent on investment from outside faced a sudden shock to their public and private sectors. This explains how Spain, for example, could go from balanced budgets to an enormously damaging economic crisis in just a few years. In the good times its government and public services benefited from the tax revenues of a growing economy, but when the inflows into the property and other sectors stopped, Spain was hit with a major economic crisis and its budget swiftly moved into deficit.

It is worth underlining that within this context of structural imbalances different countries had quite different crises. Cyprus, Greece, Ireland and Portugal fell into sovereign debt crises for different reasons, as did a number of non-Eurozone Member States. There is no simple country-level narrative of economic crisis because the Cypriot, Greek, Irish and Portuguese – let alone the Spanish, Italian, Latvian and Hungarian – economies and political systems are very different. Notably, there is no evidence that irresponsible decisions in health policy were significant in the plight of most of those countries. Even if the health system shared broader problems in public administration, no account can explain the economic crisis as a result of bad health policy and administration.

The dominant theory of the crisis among European Union decision-makers was that it was born of public policy in the debtor states. Essentially, the theory was that they exploited market expectations that Eurozone Member States would be bailed out to run fiscal or macroeconomic imbalances (or, less judgmentally, that they faced no constraints in irresponsible borrowing because the markets failed to price their risk of default correctly). There are other theories of what went wrong,[6] but the theory that post-crisis EU fiscal governance was built around was that the causes of the crisis could have been addressed by Member States had their governments been given suitable incentives, and that future crises could be avoided if Member States were given different incentives.

---

6   The best explanations find little support for the idea that overspending governments were to blame and instead focus on structural internal imbalances within the Eurozone and the flow of speculative capital. *See* Pérez SA (2019). A Europe of creditor and debtor states: explaining the north/south divide in the Eurozone. *West European Politics*, 42(5):989–1014; Johnston A, Regan A (2016). European monetary integration and the incompatibility of national varieties of capitalism. *JCMS: Journal of Common Market Studies*, 54(2):318–36; Johnston A (2016). *From convergence to crisis: labor markets and the instability of the Euro*. Cornell University Press; Johnston A, Hancké B, Pant S (2014). Comparative institutional advantage in the European sovereign debt crisis. *Comparative Political Studies*, 47(13):1771–800; Dyson K (2012). 'Maastricht Plus': Managing the Logic of Inherent Imperfections. *Journal of European Integration*, 34(7):791–808. These authors do not agree completely with one another, but they are united in finding little or no support for the theory that it was self-indulgent public policy in debtor states that caused the crisis.

In the midst of the 2010 crisis, the solution European leaders arrived at was a mixture of short-term and longer-term measures designed to reduce "moral hazard" (irresponsible lending due to expectations of a bailout) due to "soft budget constraints" (budget constraints that were not really binding due to expectations of a bailout). The idea was to arrange bailout mechanisms at the same time as making budget constraints for EU Member States harder and more effective. The logic was partly an effort to address the crisis and its underlying roots, and partly a political response to outrage in creditor countries at the size of the bailouts they were supporting.

The short-term solution was conditional loans to the countries in the biggest crisis, administered by a Troika of the European Commission, the European Central Bank and the International Monetary Fund (IMF).[7] The loans allowed the countries under the Troika's jurisdiction to continue to pay their bondholders. The loans came with conditions. Conditionality in these circumstances means that the loan carries policy and fiscal targets, and is disbursed as the debtor country hits those targets. It is a common tool that international financial institutions, including the IMF, have used extensively around the world. The theory behind conditional loans is that they directly improve policy so that the country will recover and not enter another crisis later. Indirectly, conditional loans make a bailout even more unpleasant and therefore deter reliance on future bailouts.[8]

The conditional loans were paired with the establishment of a stronger set of fiscal governance mechanisms that were intended to prevent future bad behaviour. This is the fiscal governance system discussed in section 5.2 below. Essentially, the idea is to harden budget constraints in a variety of ways: by monitoring Member State finances and economies more closely, by tying penalties such as fines and loss of EU support to prudent policy, by hardening budget rules in domestic law and constitutions, and by making it clear that support from the ECB and the rest of the EU in a crisis depends on a history of demonstrably prudent policy.

The core weakness of the entire logic is that it treats the Eurozone as the sum of its parts: if every Member State were equally prudent, runs the logic, then the whole Eurozone would be stable. The problem is that while individual EU Member States are relatively small, open economies, the size of the EU as a whole makes it a large and relatively closed economy more comparable to the United States than to any individual EU Member State. The different EU Member States run long-term surpluses between one another which appear to

---

7   Sokol T, Mijatović N (2017). "EU health law and policy and the Eurozone crisis", in Hervey, T, Young C & Bishop L (eds.). *Research Handbook on EU Health Law and Policy*. Cheltenham: Edward Elgar Publishing, pp. 291–313.

8   Fahy N (2012). Who is shaping the future of European health systems? *BMJ*, 344:e1712; Greer S (2014). Structural adjustment comes to Europe: lessons for the Eurozone from the conditionality debates. *Global Social Policy*, 14(1):51–71.

be structural and which have no obvious solution in current EU law and policy, since a state with an external payments surplus is generally viewed as successful even if that surplus is some other Member State's destabilizing deficit. The new system's overall effectiveness has not yet been tested by a serious economic downturn, but it is not clear that the fiscal governance system of the EU today, which is based on enforcing Member State prudence, is able to address Europe-wide systemic problems.

5.2   Fiscal governance

The fiscal governance system developed in the aftermath of the debt crisis focuses on ensuring that Member States will adopt policies compliant with the Stability and Growth Pact (SGP) and do not create the kinds of macroeconomic imbalances that allowed Spain or Ireland to be perfectly compliant with the SGP in 2008 but face enormous crises when their property and banking bubbles burst in 2010. It has three principal legal components, which we discuss briefly here. The previous edition of this book provides a more detailed analysis of the legal arrangements, and readers are encouraged to consult it.[9]

5.2.1   Strengthened fiscal governance in the EU: the six-pack and the two-pack

The 2011 and 2013 reforms of the SGP – known respectively as the "six-pack"[10] and the "two-pack"[11] – were the EU's response to the high and rising debt levels seen in a number of Member States both within and outside the Eurozone. The six-pack reforms are appropriately named. They considerably toughen the SGP both by making corrective measures such as fines easier to apply and by increasing the authority of the Commission to monitor the economies and

---

9   Greer SL et al. (2014). *Everything You Always Wanted to Know About European Union Health Policy But Were Afraid to Ask*. First edition. Copenhagen: WHO Regional office for Europe, on behalf of the European Observatory on Health Systems and Policies.

10   The six-pack: *European Parliament and Council (2011). Regulation (EU) No. 1175/2011 of 16 November 2011 amending Council Regulation (EC) No. 1466/97 on the strengthening of the surveillance of budgetary positions and the surveillance and coordination of economic policies, Council Regulation (EU) No. 1177/2011 of 8 November 2011 amending Regulation (EC) No. 1467/97 on speeding up and clarifying the implementation of the excessive deficit procedure, Regulation (EU) No. 1173/2011 of 16 November 2011 on the effective enforcement of budgetary surveillance in the euro area, Council Directive 2011/85/EU of 8 November 2011 on requirements for budgetary frameworks of the Member States, Council Directive 2011/85/EU of 8 November 2011 on requirements for budgetary frameworks of the Member States, Regulation (EU) No. 1176/2011 of 16 November 2011 on the prevention and correction of macroeconomic imbalances*. Luxembourg: Publications Office of the European Union.

11   The two-pack: European Parliament and Council (2013). *Regulation (EU) No. 473/2013 on common provisions for monitoring and assessing draft budgetary plans and ensuring the correction of excessive deficit of the Member States in the euro area, Regulation 472/2013 on the strengthening of economic and budgetary surveillance of Member States in the euro area experiencing or threatened with serious difficulties with respect to their financial stability*. Luxembourg: Publications Office of the European Union.

budget decisions of Member States. The two-pack reforms built on the six-pack reforms by requiring States to provide more information to the Commission for monitoring purposes.

The reformed SGP now has two arms: a preventive arm and a corrective arm. The SGP's preventive arm was established by Article 121 of the TFEU and was designed to "ensure that fiscal policy is conducted in a sustainable manner" by establishing a cycle of economic and budgetary monitoring and assessment.[12] States are expected to make progress towards predefined objectives, with this progress assessed during an annual review process called the European Semester (*see* section 5.3).

Stability Programmes and Convergence Programmes are terms used to describe the outlines of medium-term budget plans that are compiled by Member States.[13] They are submitted and assessed annually under the European Semester process. Stability Programmes are submitted by Eurozone States, while Convergence Programmes, which also contain monetary strategies, are submitted by non-Eurozone States. Stability and Convergence Programmes are used to put forward medium-term objectives: country-specific, medium-term budgetary objectives defined in terms of a state's structural budget balance.[14]

The SGP's corrective arm is established by Article 126 of the TFEU and centres around the Excessive Deficit Procedure (EDP). The EDP is designed to ensure that Member States comply with the deficit and debt rules as defined in the TFEU.[15] Despite keeping its name, the EDP was expanded through the 2011 reforms and is now used to enforce both rules. The procedure can be invoked if

---

12 European Commission (2013). *EU economic governance: stability and growth pact.* Brussels: European Commission. Available at: http://ec.europa.eu/economy_finance/economic_governance/sgp/, accessed 14 July 2014.

13 European Commission (2013). *Multilateral economic coordination and surveillance.* Brussels: European Commission. Available at: http://ec.europa.eu/economy_finance/economic_governance/sgp/convergence/, accessed 14 July 2014.

14 "The actual *budget balance* net of the *cyclical component and one-off and other temporary measures.* The structural balance gives a measure of the underlying trend in the budget balance." European Commission (2013). *EU economic governance: stability and growth pact glossary.* Brussels: European Commission. Available at: http://ec.europa.eu/economy_finance/economic_governance/sgp/glossary_en.htm, accessed 14 July 2014; on the complexities of calculation involved in the new fiscal governance, see Mabbett D, Schelkle W (2016). "Searching under the lamppost", in Caporaso J & Rhodes M (eds.). *Political and Economic Dynamics of the Eurozone Crisis.* Oxford: Oxford University Press, pp. 122–44.

15 The Maastricht reference values are defined in the TFEU, Protocol 12; A "satisfactory rate of debt reduction is reduction by 1/20th annually on average taken over a period of three years". This is known as the 1/20 rule. *See* European Commission (2011). Press release: European governance six-pack enters into force (MEMO/11/898). Brussels: European Commission. Available at: http://europa.eu/rapid/press-release_MEMO-11-898_en.htm, accessed 14 July 2014.

one or both of the rules is broken, with the same procedure used for debt and deficit breaches (with some exceptions).[16]

Under the EDP, the Commission monitors Member States' financial status. If the Commission decides that a Member State has breached or is at risk of breaching a rule or both rules, the EDP begins. The Commission informs the Member State and the Council. Exceptions can be granted for Member States that have faced events outside their control, such as natural disaster or severe economic downturn, but only if the excess over the deficit/debt is close to the threshold and considered to be temporary.

The Council decides if an excessive deficit exists. If the answer is yes, the Commission proposes and the Council adopts recommendations to correct the situation. These recommendations are not made public unless the Council thinks that the Member State has not responded according to the agreed timetable (usually six months, or three for severe cases).

If the Member State does not comply with the recommendations, a range of actions can be taken by the Council. The Council can require the Member State concerned to publish additional information, to be specified by the Council, before issuing bonds and securities; can invite the EIB to reconsider its lending policy towards the Member State concerned; can require the Member State concerned to make a non-interest-bearing deposit of an appropriate size with the EU until the excessive deficit has been corrected; or can impose fines.

These changes certainly make the "corrective" elements of the SGP more stringent. But the real surprise for observers is that there are also strict penalties for non-compliance under the preventive arm, including the requirement to lodge an interest-bearing deposit of 0.2% of GDP, which, if non-compliance continues, can turn into an annual fine, and the possible suspension of Cohesion Fund money until the excessive deficit is corrected.

5.2.2 The Treaty on Coordination, Stability and Governance

Many of the EU's core policies and principles are subsequently enshrined in treaty law as a way to bolster their legitimacy.[17] In the case of the six-pack, however, the treaty in question is not primary EU law. The Treaty on Stability, Coordination and Governance in the Economic and Monetary Union (TSCG) is a non-EU international treaty signed by 25 Member States in 2012. The TSCG contains

16 European Commission (2013). *European economic governance: the corrective arm*. Brussels: European Commission. Available at: http://ec.europa.eu/economy_finance/economic_governance/sgp/corrective_arm/index_en.htm. accessed 14 July 2014.

17 European Commission (2012). *Economic and financial affairs. Six-pack? Two-pack? Fiscal compact? A short guide to the new EU fiscal governance*. Brussels: European Commission. Available at: http://ec.europa.eu/economy_finance/articles/governance/2012-03-14_six_pack_en.htm, accessed 14 July 2014.

the Fiscal Compact and is sometimes referred to as the Fiscal Compact Treaty. The TSCG is binding on Eurozone States, while other Member States can choose to be bound once they adopt the euro or can choose provisions they wish to comply with before euro adoption. The TSCG entered into force in 2013 after 12 States ratified it.[18] It was not signed by the United Kingdom or the Czech Republic and pre-dates Croatia's EU membership. That is why, despite its stated intent to be part of enhanced cooperation under EU law and to become part of the treaties themselves, it is currently a separate international agreement.

As a result, the six-pack and the TSCG run in parallel, although their main normative elements do closely relate to one another.[19] In some ways, the TSCG mirrors the content of the EU's economic governance. The TSCG requires the contracted States to converge towards the medium-term objectives they have defined under the SGP, and it re-states the SGP's debt rule. The TSCG also mimics RQMV by committing contracting States to vote in support of the Commission when determining excessive deficits. The definitions of what constitutes a significant deviation from the rules and exceptional circumstances are the same.

In other ways, however, the TSCG goes beyond EU law. Contracting States are committed to a lower deficit ceiling than under the SGP: 1% of GDP for States with debt below 60% of GDP, and 0.5% for those with debt above 60% of GDP. States are committed to transposing their commitments, including their medium-term objectives, into national law of a "binding force and permanent character, preferably constitutional". Correction must be put in place to ensure that action is taken when a State deviates from a path that will ensure the achievement of the medium-term objective. Instead of the Council and the Commission, the CJEU can issue a ruling requiring States to implement the new rules and can impose a financial sanction amounting to 0.1% of GDP if the State fails to comply with the ruling. Compliance with the agreement is supposed to be monitored by new independent institutions at the national level, under guidelines issued by the Commission to govern their creation.

The TSCG is not all stick and no carrot, however. The carrot in question is the new European Stability Mechanism, a consolidated Europe-wide fund that provides financial assistance to contracting States. From March 2013 the TSCG limits access to financial assistance through the European Stability Mechanism

---

18 The TSCG has now been ratified in the following countries: Austria, Cyprus, Denmark, Estonia, Finland, France, Germany, Greece, Hungary, Ireland, Italy, Latvia, Lithuania, Luxembourg, Malta, the Netherlands, Poland, Portugal, Romania, Slovakia, Slovenia, Spain and Sweden.

19 European Commission (2012). *Economic and financial affairs; does the fiscal compact succeed the six-pack or does it run alongside it?* Brussels: European Commission. Available at: http://ec.europa.eu/economy_finance/ articles/governance/2012-03-14_six_pack_en.htm, accessed 14 July 2014.

(replacing the European Financial Stabilizing Mechanism) to countries that have enacted the TSCG.

5.3 The European Semester

The European Semester is the main vehicle for the formulation of goals and surveillance of public policies in the EU. It is based on the six-pack and two-pack and draws on a long legacy of EU initiatives in public policy surveillance and coordination, such as the BEPG and the Open Method of Coordination, so it is not entirely innovative, but it is arguably much more important. In particular, the Semester's remit is anything that might affect SGP compliance or macroeconomic imbalances, and so it is effectively the open invitation to engage in detailed discussion of health policy that the treaties previously lacked.

5.3.1 The European Semester: process

The European Semester was first introduced in 2011 as part of the six-pack. It is a powerful tool for achieving consistent policy recommendations – not just among Member States, but also horizontally across EU and European programmes as well – as through the Semester the Commission can review a raft of information that is pertinent to the TSCG, Euro Plus Pact and Europe 2020, as well as the SGP and the Macroeconomic Imbalance Procedure (MIP).

The name European Semester refers to the idea that European surveillance of national budgets should come before national surveillance, which occurs during the National Semester in the second half of the year. This process is referred to as "upstream policy coordination" by the Commission[20] but has caused many to question whether the European Semester leaves national parliaments out in the cold.

The European Semester starts in October, when Member States are required to submit their draft budgets to the Commission.[21] These draft budget documents are published. The Commission can ask for redrafts if it considers that a budget plan is out of line with the SGP. In November the Commission sets out the EU's budgetary priorities for the next year through a series of reports. The first

---

20 European Commission (2013). *Economic and financial affairs: the European Semester*. Brussels: European Commission. Available at: http://ec.europa.eu/economy_finance/economic_governance/the_european_semester/index_en.htm, accessed 14 July 2014.

21 The following text draws heavily on European Commission (2013). *Economic and financial affairs: the European Semester*. Brussels: European Commission. Available at: http://ec.europa.eu/economy_finance/economic_governance/the_european_semester/index_en.htm, accessed 14 July 2014; European Commission (2013). *Making it happen: the European Semester*. Brussels: European Commission. Available at: http://ec.europa.eu/europe2020/making-it-happen/, accessed 14 July 2014; and Council of the European Union (2013). *What is the European Semester?* Brussels: Council of the European Union. Available at: http://www.consilium.europa.eu/special-reports/european-semester, accessed 14 July 2014.

key report is the Annual Growth Survey, which sets out proposed priorities. (It is reminiscent of the state of the global economy reports produced by bodies such as the OECD and the IMF.) The second key report is the Alert Mechanism Report, which flags up macroeconomic imbalances in Member States as required by the MIP and explains which Member States will subsequently be subject to in-depth review. These recommendations are discussed by the Council and the European Parliament in the following months.

These Commission reports are key agenda-setting documents. In March the European Council adopts "economic priorities" for the EU, working from the Commission's recommendations in the Annual Growth Survey. And in April Member States submit the Stability Programmes (fiscal plans drawn up by Eurozone States) or Convergence Programmes (fiscal plans drawn up by non-Eurozone States) required by the SGP, as well as the National Reform Programmes required within the Europe 2020 strategy. The Commission then publishes its in-depth reviews.

From these data, and from the rest of its ongoing surveillance, the Commission proposes a CSR for each Member State. The CSRs are endorsed by the European Council, discussed by the employment, economic and finance, and competitiveness councils, and then adopted by the DG for Economic and Financial Affairs (ECFIN).

The European Semester is a vital link between the soft-law style of target setting often associated with the EU's new governance mechanisms, such as Europe 2020, and the harder structural adjustment politics of the EU's economic crisis. By beginning with budgetary discipline and structural adjustment issues, from the legal basis that these issues have in the TFEU and the normative basis that they have in ECFIN, the European Semester exists as a framework that can impose its hierarchy on other, non-economic policy areas. So now it is not just a framework for economic policy governance, it is also a framework for social and policy governance in a way that its predecessors never really became. This becomes clear when the relationship between the European Semester and the soft-law governance tools such as Europe 2020 and the Euro Plus Pact are considered.

Each Member State's Europe 2020 commitments are articulated via a National Reform Programme, a report stating the policy measures to be adopted by the State and explaining how they meet that State's EU-level targets – stemming from both the Europe 2020 strategy and other initiatives including the CSRs and Euro Plus Pact commitments. These National Reform Programmes are reviewed by the Commission during the European Semester, alongside their economic governance equivalents, the Stability and Convergence Programmes.

Commitments made under the Euro Plus Pact are treated in a similar manner. The Euro Plus Pact, also known as the Competitiveness Pact or the Pact for the Euro, is an agreement reached in March 2011 by 23 Member States, as reported in the conclusions of the European Council.[22] Interestingly, as well as the Eurozone countries, the Pact includes six non-Eurozone countries: Bulgaria, Denmark, Latvia, Lithuania, Poland and Romania. These countries agreed to adopt targets in four broad areas of policy, including labour market and employment reforms, competitiveness, fiscal policy and financial stability measures. The Pact is designed to be flexible, and not all Member States have made pledges in each of these areas. Where these pledges do exist, they vary in their specificity: from adopting a fiscal rule to increasing labour participation of certain demographic groups.

Unlike its hard-law siblings, the Euro Plus Pact was agreed to under the OMC. There is consequently very little infrastructure supporting it and little public documentation. It also means that the European Parliament has no formal role in scrutinizing activities under the Pact.[23] Like the Europe 2020 targets, pledges made under the Pact are monitored through the European Semester process, with Member States publicly stating that there needed to be consistency rather than overlap between the Euro Plus Pact and the information presented in National Reform, Stability and Convergence Programmes. To that end, Member States urged a focus on fewer, high-impact measures that combine "durable consolidation of public finances with structural reforms".[24]

5.3.2 The European Semester: health policy content

The power of the Semester, legally and politically, rests not in its contribution to health and well-being but in its contribution to the EU's fiscal governance. Legally, the policy instruments underlying it are grounded in fiscal rules, not social or health policy objectives. Politically, it was instituted to solve problems of moral hazard and soft budget constraints, not to improve social or health policy.

As might have been expected, the Semester process therefore began in a way that was worrisome from a health and healthcare perspective. Organizationally, the initial key directorates-general were Employment, Taxation (TAXUD), and, very much pre-eminent, Economic and Financial Affairs (ECFIN). The Council formation overseeing it and making the ultimate decisions was ECOFIN, the Council of Finance Ministers. From some perspectives, it was essentially a vehicle

---

22 The following draws on European Commission (2011). *Background on the Euro Plus Pact*. Brussels: European Commission. Available at: http://ec.europa.eu/europe2020/pdf/euro_plus_pact_background_december_2011_en.pdf, accessed 14 July 2014.

23 Library of the European Parliament (2012). *Library Briefing: Parliament's role in anti-crisis decision-making*. Brussels: Library of the European Parliament.

24 Council of the European Union (2012). *Euro Plus Pact: the way forward – conclusions of Member States participating in the Euro Plus Pact*. Brussels: Council of the European Union.

for a network of finance ministries to tighten their control over key areas of revenue and expenditure such as health.[25]

The initial Semester CSRs reflected this political, legal and organizational focus on fiscal sustainability as understood by finance ministries.[26] There were initially relatively few health-related CSRs and they were often either fairly crude or amounted to an EU endorsement of existing Member State plans (as happened especially clearly with Austria, whose CSRs in the first years mirrored quite precisely the plans that the health and finance ministers had already agreed). Some CSRs were relatively inexplicable and clearly showed a lack of understanding of health policy, as with the suggestion in 2015 that France might reduce its health expenditure by increasing the number of health professionals it trained, in defiance of what is known about the importance of supply-induced demand in healthcare.

Over time, a variety of pressures began to change the Semester process and content. The process changed, with DG TAXUD less visible and DG EMPL and SANTE more visible. Under the Juncker Commission, the Secretariat-General became more important in the process, especially vis-à-vis DG ECFIN (which was headed by a Socialist from France). At the same time, a number of conflicts between Member States and the Commission led to a less clear-cut and punitive application of fiscal governance than the law alone might have suggested.

Meanwhile, after pressure from health ministers, DG SANTE, and other health policy interests, DG SANTE became a more important part of the Semester process. The EPSCO council's pressure on the Commission (section 3.5.2) led to the Commission's 2014 Communication on effective, accessible and resilient health systems, which emphasized the need to strengthen health systems and lent extra authority to participation of DG SANTE in health systems discussions. In other words, a process that was initially quite exclusive and focused on narrow fiscal policy goals was broadened out as other affected interests sought participation and other priorities were pushed onto the agenda.[27] The result was more discussion of health and healthcare, more sophisticated discussion of health and healthcare, and more sensitive policy recommendations. The effects are visible now, when it can seem plausible to see the Semester as an evolution of the OMC as much as an instrument for fiscal control.

25 Stamati F, Baeten R (2015). *Healthcare Reforms and the Crisis*. Brussels: European Trade Union Institute.
26 Azzopardi-Muscat N et al. (2015). EU Country Specific Recommendations for Health Systems in the European Semester Process: Trends, Discourse and Predictors. *Health Policy*, 119:375–83.
27 Greer SL, Brooks E (2020). Termites of Solidarity in the House of Austerity. University of Michigan, working paper. For a review of the health and equity dimensions of the Semester, with case studies, and suggestions for further improvement, *see* EuroHealthNet "The European Semester 2019 from a health equity perspective" 2019. https://eurohealthnet.eu/sites/eurohealthnet.eu/files/publications/FINAL%20 The%20European%20Semester%202019%20from%20a%20health%20equity%20perspective.pdf, accessed 27 September 2019.

Box 5.1 lists the formal recommendations for 2019 as agreed by the Council. In most cases a country with a recommendation has a paragraph-long discussion in the text summarizing some key healthcare issues and challenges (some of which is quoted in the box). The apparent vagueness of some recommendations is therefore balanced in some cases by more precision in the text (Box 5.2). Some countries have neither recommendations nor discussion in the text, which presumably means that no attribute of their healthcare policies has been deemed a threat to fiscal sustainability.

What should stand out from these recommendations is just how far they have come from the institutionalized austerity of the early Semester. In case after case, the equity, effectiveness and quality of the healthcare system are raised as issues. This is a much subtler and more health-informed approach than was seen in the early years of the Semester, and one that values a broader range of outcomes and appreciates the logic of longer-term investments. It is evidence of a process of "socialization" that scholars have noted.[28] Thus we can see that countries such as Latvia and Lithuania are given advice to improve the quality and affordability of their health systems, and Italy to redress its regional inequalities, while Cyprus and Ireland receive endorsement of their moves towards universal health coverage (with a particularly supportive discussion of the Irish policy challenge: *see* Box 5.1) Member State ownership is in general a value in the Semester process as it operates now, which effectively means that the Commission tries to avoid recommendations that lack support within the Member State.[29] Compared to the earlier handling of health in CSRs, this is a dramatic difference.

Another point that is visible in the recommendations for several countries (Austria, Ireland, Malta, Portugal and Slovenia) is the linkage between the fiscal sustainability of the healthcare system and that of the long-term care and pension systems. The recommendation is often concretely about reducing pension liabilities, but the linkage of pensions and health is made because both are seen as costs of an ageing population. Notably, health is discussed more in these cases as a cost that will increase with ageing, like pensions, rather than an investment in reducing the costs and increasing the benefits such as informal care associated with an ageing population.

As this book went to press, incoming Commission President Ursula von der Leyen told the Parliament that she would "refocus our European Semester to make sure

---

28 Zeitlin J, Verdun A (eds.) (2018). *EU Socio-Economic Governance since the Crisis. The European Semester in Theory and Practice*. Abingdon: Routledge; Zeitlin J, Vanhercke B (2018). Socializing the European Semester: EU social and economic policy co-ordination in crisis and beyond. *Journal of European Public Policy*, 25(2):149–74.

29 Tkalec I (2019). The Council's Amendments to the Country-Specific Recommendations: More than just Cosmetics? *Journal of Contemporary European Research*, 15(2):212–27. Available at: https://doi.org/10.30950/jcer.v15i2.1001.

that we stay on track with our Sustainable Development Goals"[30] (*see* Box 2.6). This statement, along with other statements such as the Council statement on the economy of well-being (Box 1.4), suggests that the Semester, and perhaps broader EU policy, will develop a more social and coherent framework.

5.4 Structural funds

Right from the start, the EU had the objective of reducing the inequalities in development between different regions in the EU. As new countries have joined the EU over the decades, the disparities between the richest and poorest regions have also grown; alongside this, the resources allocated by the EU into countering those disparities have also grown. This should be kept in perspective; as outlined in section 5.3 on the EU budget, investment through these funds still represents only around a half of 1% of the total wealth of the EU (for 2014–2020). Nevertheless, this is still tens of billions of euros a year, is new money not tied up in existing commitments and can make a real difference when focused on particular topics and areas in the poorer countries of the EU. Because of the size of the structural funds overall, it means that the actual amounts invested from the structural funds compares well with the other major health-specific funds for health research and are much larger than those from the specific programme for health.[31]

There are three main structural funds:

The European Regional Development Fund (ERDF).   This finances direct aid to companies to create sustainable jobs, infrastructure development, financial instruments (e.g. local development funds) and technical assistance.

The European Social Fund (ESF).   This is the "human resources" fund, focusing on worker adaptation (e.g. retraining of workers from declining industries), employment and social integration.

The Cohesion Fund.   This is particularly focused on the poorer Member States – in particular the ten eastern European countries (Bulgaria, the Czech Republic, Estonia, Hungary, Latvia, Lithuania, Poland, Romania, Slovakia and Slovenia). Examples of funding include trans-European transport networks and environment-related projects in particular.

---

30 Ursula von der Leyen (2019). "A Union that strives for more. Political guidelines for the next European Commission 2019–2024". Available at: https://www.europarl.europa.eu/resources/library/media/2019 0716RES57231/20190716RES57231.pdf.

31 Watson J (2009). *Health and structural funds in 2007–2013: country and regional assessment.* Brussels: DG Health and Consumer Protection. Available at: http://ec.europa.eu/health/health_structural_funds/docs/watson_report.pdf, accessed 14 July 2014.

Box 5.1 *2019 Country Specific Recommendations with reference to health*

Where there is substantial text discussion of the healthcare system but no health-related recommendations, some of the text is excerpted.

Austria: Ensure the sustainability of the health, long-term care, and pension systems, including by adjusting the statutory retirement age in view of expected gains in life expectancy.

Belgium: No recommendations.

Bulgaria: Improve access to health services, including by reducing out-of-pocket payments and addressing shortages of health professionals.

Croatia: No recommendations.

Cyprus: Take measures to ensure that the National Health System becomes operational in 2020, as planned, while preserving its long-term sustainability.

Czech Republic: No recommendations.

Denmark: No recommendations.

Estonia: No recommendations. (Noted in text: "challenges point to the need to deliver affordable and good quality social and healthcare services in an integrated way and to develop a comprehensive long-term care framework".)

Finland: No recommendations.

France: No recommendations. (Noted in text: the overall fiscal targeting's "success will depend on meeting planned expenditure targets defined for the central and local governments and for the healthcare system".)

Germany: No recommendations.

Greece: Focus investment-related economic policy on sustainable transport and logistics, environmental protection, energy efficiency, renewable energy and interconnection projects, digital technologies, research and development, education, skills, employability, health, and the renewal of urban areas, taking into account regional disparities and the need to ensure social inclusion.

Hungary: Improve health outcomes by supporting preventive health measures and strengthening primary healthcare.

Ireland: Address the expected increase in age-related expenditure by making the healthcare system more cost-effective and by fully implementing pension reform plans. (A longer text discussion notes that "The planned reform represents a credible vision for making the health system universally accessible and sustainable, meeting the demands of an ageing population and shifting care into the community, with a stronger focus on prevention. This is likely to have a positive impact in reducing the reliance on acute care, thereby making healthcare more cost-effective. However, implementation is endangered by the health system's difficulties in addressing the duplicate health insurance market and effectively managing its own budget, performance and workforce in the short term.")

Italy: No recommendations. (Noted in text: "The outcome of the health system overall is good, despite below-EU average spending. Nevertheless, the provision of healthcare largely varies across regions, affecting access, equity and efficiency, and could be improved through better administration and by monitoring the delivery of standard levels of services.")

Latvia: Increase the accessibility, quality and cost-effectiveness of the healthcare system.

Lithuania: Increase the quality, affordability and efficiency of the healthcare system.

Luxembourg: No recommendations.

Malta: Ensure the fiscal sustainability of the healthcare and pension systems, including by restricting early retirement and adjusting the statutory retirement age in view of expected gains in life expectancy.

Netherlands: No recommendations.

Poland: Focus investment-related economic policy on innovation, transport, notably on its sustainability, digital and energy infrastructure, healthcare and cleaner energy, taking into account regional disparities.

Portugal: No recommendations. (Noted in text: "Portugal's public finances are under continuous pressure from adverse demographic trends, notably the ageing population, with negative consequences, especially for the sustainability of the pension and health systems.")

Romania: Improve access to and cost-efficiency of healthcare, including through the shift to outpatient care.

Slovakia: Achieve the medium-term budgetary objective in 2020. Safeguard the long-term sustainability of public finances, notably that of the healthcare and pension systems. Focus investment-related economic policy on healthcare, research and innovation, transport, notably on its sustainability, digital infrastructure, energy efficiency, competitiveness of small and medium-sized enterprises, and social housing, taking into account regional disparities.

Slovenia: Adopt and implement reforms in healthcare and long-term care that ensure quality, accessibility and long-term fiscal sustainability.

Spain: No recommendations.

Sweden: No recommendations.

United Kingdom: No recommendations.

Source: https://ec.europa.eu/info/publications/2019-european-semester-country-specific-recommendations-council-recommendations_en.

Box 5.2 *How to read Semester documents*

A Semester Country Specific Recommendation is both a legal document and a major statement of priorities since there are far more policy issues than there are opportunities for CSRs. As Box 5.1 shows, recommendations can often be somewhat opaque on their own. What, exactly, does it mean that in 2019 Lithuania was advised to "Increase the quality, affordability and efficiency of the healthcare system?" The answer in these cases is to work backwards. First, consult the "recitals" – the long section at the top of the CSRs that explains the rationale and context. Paragraph 12 of the Commission's proposed CSRs explains:

"Weak health outcomes and low investment in healthcare are persisting challenges. There remains significant potential to rationalise the use of resources through a further shift from inpatient to outpatient care. The consumption of hospital services continues to be high, with high rates of hospitalisations for chronic diseases coupled with relatively low bed occupancy rates. Further rationalisation of hospital resources use, together with targeted investments to strengthen primary care services, including in the healthcare workforce, are necessary to drive efficiency gains and improve health outcomes. The quality of care remains one of the main reasons for poor health outcomes. Measures to improve the quality of care are fragmented, with very low take-up of accreditation in the primary care sector and a lack of application of the accreditation system in hospitals. Investment in disease prevention measures is particularly low. Moreover, steps taken to strengthen disease prevention measures at local level lack an overarching vision and are impaired by a lack of systemic co-operation between public health offices and primary care. Lastly, low levels of health spending coupled with relatively high informal payments and high out-of-pocket payments have negative implications for equity of access to healthcare."

The evidence base for this analysis, as with most such analyses in the Semester, is in the Country Report (in this case published as Commission Staff Working Document SWD (2019) 1014, published alongside the CSRs). It has extensive discussions of the state of Lithuanian health and health policies. Its presence reflects the general agreement that health is an issue with consequences for the Lithuanian fiscal and economic profile, as well as its social rights and protection. The evidence base and intellectual structure of the discussion of health is rooted one step further back, in the State of Health in the EU report on Lithuania, which is part of the series jointly produced with the OECD and the European Observatory on Health Systems and Policies and which brings together evidence from the larger health research field (3.6.1).

The process of feeding information into the Semester can be read in reverse, as a funnel whose widest part is the State of Health in the EU Country Health Profiles, narrowing to the discussion of health in the Country Reports, and then narrowing further to the recitals of the CSRs, and ending in the sentence that makes up a normal CSR. At each stage there are consultations within the Commission and with Member States, as well as with at least some interested parties in the Member States. (Member States have great influence over which parties can engage with the Commission, e.g. some decline to let regional governments and the Commission interact in Semester discussions.)

There are also other smaller instruments addressing specific priorities at European level (i.e. technical assistance to the "new" Member States in preparing projects, access to finance for small to medium-sized enterprises, urban investment and microfinance). The EU Solidarity Fund is a separate emergency assistance fund in the event of major natural disasters.

In principle, structural funds are part of the Semester, and Member States that seriously violate the rules of fiscal governance should have their access to funds reduced. In practice, and perhaps unsurprisingly, Member States and EU institutions alike prefer to compromise and soften the relevant fiscal governance rules.[32]

Historically, the use of the structural funds has reflected a fairly conservative model of economic growth, focusing on major infrastructure projects and not prioritizing "softer" sectors such as health. However, in recent years there has been somewhat greater recognition of the potential economic contribution of investing in health and healthcare.[33] Indeed, during the last programming period (2014–2020), there were health-related projects in 27 Member States. Geographically, this investment is focused on eastern European countries. Specific investment to improve and modernize health infrastructure has been included in the programmes for Bulgaria, the Czech Republic, Greece, Hungary, Latvia, Lithuania, Poland, Romania and Slovakia. Modernization of information systems and increased use of e-health has also been a priority in the new Member States, as has (to a lesser extent) human resources investment. However, there has also been investment from the structural funds in the health systems of western Europe, including in France, Germany, Greece, Italy, Portugal and Spain. Health systems can also benefit from investment by the structural funds in other sectors, such as in knowledge hubs, innovation clusters or in more general improvement in community facilities.

---

32 Sacher M (2019). Macroeconomic Conditionalities: Using the Controversial Link between EU Cohesion Policy and Economic Governance. *Journal of Contemporary European Research*, 15(2):179–93. Available at: https://doi.org/10.30950/jcer.v15i2.1005. For why it should not be surprising, *see* Kleine M (2013). *Informal governance in the European Union: How governments make international organizations work*. Ithaca: Cornell University Press.

33 Suhrcke M et al. (2005). *The contribution of health to the economy in the European Union*. Luxembourg: Publications Office of the European Union.

One striking example is Hungary, which made the most use of any Member State of the structural funds for health during the 2007–2013 period.[34] Over this period, the Hungarian authorities decided to allocate €1.8 billion of the structural funding to healthcare infrastructure projects.[35] This covered a wide range of projects, in particular the inpatient care sector (accounting for over 75% of funding). In fact, the structural funds have become the principal source of capital investment for the Hungarian health system. The detailed priorities of expenditure have changed somewhat under different governments during the programme period. Regional operational programmes have supported specific adaptations in different parts of the country, in particular strengthening primary care through developing local health centres as well as establishing independent outpatient centres.

This represents both good news and bad news. The good news is that it is entirely possible to justify health-related expenditure under the structural funds, and a wide range of health expenditure at that. The bad news is that this expenditure has to be justified in terms of wider objectives than health alone – something that historically the health sector has not always been effective at doing. The European Commission's 2013 Staff Working Paper on investing in health also made some specific recommendations for how the structural funds should be used by Member States to invest in health.[36] The paper recommended that Member States use the funds to best effect by:

- investing in health infrastructure that fosters a transformational change in the health system, in particular reinforcing the shift from a hospital-centred model to community-based care and integrated services;

- improving access to affordable, sustainable and high-quality healthcare, in particular with a view to reducing health inequalities between regions and giving disadvantaged groups and marginalized communities better access to healthcare;

- supporting the adaptation, up-skilling and lifelong learning of the health workforce; and

- fostering active, healthy ageing to promote employability and employment and to enable people to stay active for longer.

---

34 Dowdeswell B (2011). *EUREGIO III Case study: Hungary structural fund programme development and management 2007/13*. Brussels: EUREGIO III. Available at: EUREGIO III Case study – Hungary.pdf, accessed 14 July 2014.

35 Gaál P et al. (2011). Hungary: Health system review. *Health Systems in Transition*, 13(5):1–266.

36 European Commission (2013). *Staff Working Document SWD(2013)43: investing in health*. Brussels: European Commission.

Table 5.1   *Health-related actions in the proposed thematic objectives*

Health-related actions	Which thematic objective?	Which fund?
Development of small to medium-sized enterprises reflecting new societal demands or products and services linked to the ageing population, care and health	3. Competitiveness of small and medium-sized enterprises	ERDF
Access to employment, including long-term employment opportunities created by structural shifts in the labour market, such as the care and health sectors	8. Promoting employment and supporting labour mobility	ESF
New business creation in sectors including care and health, including self-employment and entrepreneurship for young people	8. Promoting employment and supporting labour mobility	ESF, ERDF
Integrated employability measures including access to health services.	9. Promoting social inclusion and combating poverty	ESF
Modernization to improve the cost–effectiveness and adequacy of healthcare and social services	9. Promoting social inclusion and combating poverty	ESF
Integration of marginalized communities such as the Roma, including access to healthcare (e.g. disease prevention, health education, patient safety)	9. Promoting social inclusion and combating poverty	ESF
Specific actions targeting people with disabilities and chronic disease with a view to increasing their labour market participation, enhancing their social inclusion and reducing inequalities in terms of education attainment and health status	9. Promoting social inclusion and combating poverty	ESF
Enhancing access to affordable, sustainable and high-quality healthcare with a view to reducing health inequalities, supporting disease prevention and promoting e-health, including through targeted actions focused on particularly vulnerable groups; integrated approaches for early childhood education and care services; support for the transition from institutional care to community-based care services for children without parental care, people with disabilities, the elderly and people with mental disorders, with a focus on integration between health and social services	9. Promoting social inclusion and combating poverty	ESF
Investment in health infrastructure to improve access to health services, and to contribute to the modernization, structural transformation and sustainability of health systems, leading to measurable improvements in health outcomes, including e-health measures	9. Promoting social inclusion and combating poverty	ERDF
Capacity-building for stakeholders delivering health policies, and sectoral and territorial pacts to mobilize for reform at national, regional and local level	11. Institutional capacity-building and efficient public administration	ESF

Notes: ESF: European Social Fund; ERDF: European Regional Development Fund.

This emphasizes the importance of including health in the strategic planning for the new 2021–2027 period, by identifying key challenges, setting key health-related objectives that fit with overall strategic priorities, and identifying interventions and corresponding funding sources. Key lessons learnt about how to improve on the past are also suggested: getting in early, while wider strategies are still being set; providing evidence and data to support the proposal; and taking a broad participative approach (building a wide consensus, noting that the programming period lasts longer than individual political mandates).

The overall strategic planning for expenditure for the 2021–2027 period was under way at national and European level at the time of writing. It remains to be seen how much the Member States and the Commission will choose to make health a priority within those plans. Given the overall pressure on public budgets, and the emergence of the structural funds as the predominant source of capital investment in an increasing number of Member States, this will be critical in shaping the development of European health systems and their response to issues such as demographic ageing.

On a somewhat different track, but with great potential importance, is the possibility of adding rule of law conditionality to structural funds, discussed in Box 1.3. The Commission suggested that in the event of "generalised deficiencies" being identified in the rule of law of a Member State, "measures should include the suspension of payments and of commitments, a reduction of funding under existing commitments, and a prohibition to conclude new commitments with recipients".[37] Given the importance of structural funds, this is an important and politically contentious proposal.[38]

5.5   The European Investment Bank

Founded in 1958 and located in Luxembourg, the European Investment Bank (EIB) provides funding for projects that seek to achieve EU goals, within or outside the European Union. A wide range of health projects are eligible for EIB finance, including laboratory equipment, medical scanners, e-health digital imaging, electronic patient records and clinical decision support systems. The Bank is also increasingly financing intangible health investments, such as medical

---

37 COM(2018) 324 final, 2018/0136(COD) Proposal for a Regulation of the European Parliament and of the Council on the protection of the Union's budget in case of generalised deficiencies as regards the rule of law in the Member States.

38 Going further, there is research raising the possibility that structural funds in sufficient amounts can actually distort politics in beneficiary Member States, a variant on what political scientists know as the "resource curse". See, for example, Huliaras A, Petropoulos S (2016). European Money in Greece: In Search of the Real Impact of EU Structural Funds. *JCMS: Journal of Common Market Studies*, 54(6):1332–49.

research and development.[39] Since 2000 the EIB and the European Investment Fund (EIF) have lent about €26 billion in support of health infrastructure investments (which represents around €1.5 billion on average per year), including new constructions, renovations and new equipment. Financing varied from year to year between 2000 and 2016. In 2000 the EIB Group financed projects in the health sector up to €652 million, whereas in 2010 the total volume stood at €3.4 billion; in 2016 it was €1.2 billion.[40]

At the start of the Juncker Commission in 2014, it jointly launched the Investment Plan for Europe, better known as the "Juncker Plan" with the Commission. It was developed in response to the fallout from the economic crisis, the tight limits on member states' investments, and the limited scope of other EU instruments for expenditure. The initiative, by providing budget guarantees intended to unlock other investment, funded a large number of health projects. By 2019 it had exceeded its expenditure target, though the European Court of Auditors pointed out in March 2019 that much of the expenditure either could have been provided by the private sector or other EIB programmes.[41] It was nonetheless renewed and expanded for 2021-2027, with 13 other small funding programmes folded in.

In general, the EIB is very cautious: "its modus is to lend big and lend safe", as *Financial Times* reporters put it. That approach might help to explain why such a powerful financial instrument has been so prudently used by the finance ministers who ultimately control it and also why its shifts – the Juncker Plan and its new green focus – are relatively low-profile despite its size.[42]

39 European Investment Bank (2016). *EIB Group Support for the Social Sector*. Available at: https://www.eib.
   org/attachments/thematic/support_for_the_social_sector_en.pdf, accessed 11 June 2019.
40 Ibid. p. 3.
41 European Court of Auditors, Special report no 03/2019: European Fund for Strategic Investments: Action
   needed to make EFSI a full success. Luxembourg: European Court of Auditors.
42 Toplensky R, Barker A (2019). European Investment Bank: the EU's hidden giant. *Financial Times*, 15
   July 2019. Available at: https://www.ft.com/content/940b71f2-a3c2-11e9-a282-2df48f366f7d.

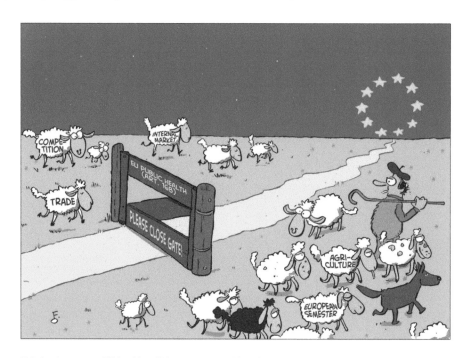

This book presents EU health policies as a gate with no fence on either side. Article 168 of the Treaty on the Functioning of the European Union (TFEU) could be seen as a gate that Member States intend to keep closed most of the time. The Article is a virtual lexicon of cautious phrases and exclusions that constrain, rather than foster, EU action in this field. With such a legal basis, it might almost seem miraculous that a considerable body of EU health policy has been developed over time. But the gate of Article 168 that Member States so laboriously constructed stands alone in a field with no fence, and so other dimensions of EU health policy and integration can simply go around it.

© Comic House/Floris Oudshoorn, reproduced with permission

Chapter 6

Conclusion

The abiding irony of EU health policy is that it is not made as a health policy in any normal sense of the term. The interests, organizations and arguments that are common in the health policy arena of the Member States are poorly represented. Instead, as discussed throughout this book, the EU's policies affecting health are made in all sorts of other ways, under all sorts of guises, and in all sorts of other venues: as fiscal governance, as environmental, labour, or social policy, or as internal market law and regulation.

6.1   The four freedoms, constitutional asymmetry and health

The three faces of EU health policy are quite different, in intention, politics, bureaucratic organization and legal base. The first face of EU health policy, discussed in chapter 1, is the closest to what health policy means in the Member States: actions taken to address causes of avoidable morbidity and mortality, whether through ensuring the safety of blood products, by developing epidemiological capacity through ECDC, by facilitating data gathering and comparison, or by supporting investments in healthcare infrastructure. These are areas in which the EU can and does take direct action to promote health. They are also the areas with the weakest policy instruments, grounded in a treaty article that is a lexicon of words used to limit EU action and which has an entire section underlining that the organization and finance of healthcare services is a competence of the Member States. The 2017 "five futures" report suggesting post-Brexit options for the EU went so far as to suggest that the EU could exist without activity in public health at all.[1] No serious report, by contrast, suggests wholly eliminating EU market integration or fiscal governance. There would be little left of the EU were that to happen.

The second face of EU health policy, market integration and regulation, is far more important and is discussed in chapter 4. It is the basis on which the EU as we know it was built, and it is the basis under which the most important policies affecting health have been made to date, including laws directly affecting healthcare on

---

1   European Commission (2017). *White Paper on the Future of Europe: Five Scenarios*.

issues such as professional mobility, patient mobility, pharmaceutical and medical devices regulation, competition law and law on state aid to industry.

The underlying *constitutional asymmetry* of the EU lies in the disjunction between these two faces, which are not equal. The ability of the EU to effect change through law, deregulation and regulation far exceeds its ability to effect change through funding or the direct provision of services. Furthermore, the principle of nondiscrimination that underlies so much European Union law and policy is best used as a tool for undoing Member State regulation through legal challenge, while reregulating that which is deregulated, through EU law, is a slow and awkward process. Member State and EU legal systems have created a large body of law and policy that deregulates, while it is legislatures and elected politicians who must re-regulate at the European level. In recent decades they have chosen to do less European re-regulation. Put another way, the EU's ability to make and correct markets is far greater than its ability to compensate for the effects of those markets.

The novelty of recent years is the third face, the dimension of EU fiscal governance. Just as the treaties provide no basis for the regulation of healthcare delivery on health grounds but permit it on the grounds of internal market law, EU law and the TSCG permit detailed attempts to regulate healthcare delivery on grounds of macroeconomic and fiscal management. It is less clear, as chapter 5 showed, just what the effect of the fiscal governance machinery will be. On one hand, its uses are becoming less clear as the initial focus on budgetary austerity has become more diffuse and other priorities have entered the Semester agenda. On the other hand, compliance with the fiscal governance system has been problematic for decades, both in terms of Member State compliance with the overall fiscal targets and in terms of the adoption of specific policy proposals. It is far from clear that the punitive arm of the fiscal governance architecture, still largely unused, will be credible or helpful in the next downturn.

Nor is it clear that the EU fiscal governance approach, which focuses on reducing imbalances and promoting budgetary rigour in each Member State, will prevent crises arising from the large internal imbalances and persistent divergences within the EU. The EU's fiscal governance system might have become more subtle and useful as a policy tool, and even given some additional health-promoting content and political force to its social policy suggestions, but there is room to doubt whether it will fulfil its key goal of preventing future crises.

6.2   Rethinking the EU health policy space

A regulatory and deregulatory approach grounded in subsidiarity and the construction of a single European market might be logically coherent and well established in practice, but it has its limits. There are multiple contradictions in the politics of EU health policy. On the one hand, surveys show popular desire for EU policies that improve health, and working for better health is an obvious way to show the citizens of Europe the benefits of the EU. On the other hand, there is very little support for a bigger EU budget or ambitious EU actions that might infringe on Member State responsibility for health policy. Likewise, the EU does much for health, but much of that is understood as something else – as environmental policy, or labour law, or health and safety law, or consumer protection law. Those actions, beneficial for health, often manifest as additional regulation which can irritate people with affected interests. The result is a set of tensions: the most effective EU actions for health are not always understood as health policies, while general popular support for EU actions to improve health collides with weak treaty bases and weaker political support for explicit EU health actions. But simply announcing that the EU will cease to emphasize public health does not solve the problem, since the EU has powerful tools to influence health that it uses in the course of regulating markets, ensuring environmental protection and health and safety, and striving for fiscal sustainability. The existence of EU policies affecting health is unavoidable. The question is whether the EU will use them explicitly for health.

In terms of health policy issues on which the EU is acting, but with questionable policy and uncertain effects, policies to do with ageing are an important issue. The third face of EU health policy, fiscal governance, is concerned about the liabilities of governments and the Semester has over various years produced repeated calls for later retirement ages and often-unspecified policy changes to ensure the fiscal sustainability of health systems (*see* section 5.2). There is scope for this debate to be more sophisticated, understanding the promotion of active and healthy ageing not just as a way to enable later retirement ages or reduce healthcare needs among older people, but as a way to invest in people across their lifecourse in order that they may make the greatest and most satisfying contribution to their own and others' lives. The Semester has become much more sophisticated in its recommendations, but it, and the EU's overall role in promoting thinking about ageing and health, could still be improved.[2]

If there were support for a stronger and more health-focused EU policy, there is legal space and a range of creative political possibilities. The State of Health in the EU is an instrument to shape the whole narrative of health policy in the EU and the Member States. One way is through direct, visible, EU health policies with output legitimacy, such as initiatives for research and action against cancer,

---

2   Cylus J, Normand C, Figueras J, 2019. *Will population ageing spell the end of the welfare state? A review of evidence and policy options.* Copenhagen:WHO Regional Office for Europe, on behalf of the European Observatory on Health Systems and Policies; and Greer SL et al. (forthcoming). *The politics of ageing and Health* (provisional title). Cambridge: Cambridge University Press.

antimicrobial resistance or the communicable diseases that climate change is bringing back to Europe. Another is through the utilization of powerful EU powers that are not part of Article 168 but name health. Public concern about chemicals and about the safety of the food system is important across Europe, as is public health concern for the effects of contemporary diets. These are core areas of EU competence and activity, especially in veterinary, agricultural, environmental protection, chemical regulation and food safety issues, and there is great scope for EU leadership should the key political interests align. Likewise, EU law affecting the economy and labour is a powerful force, with consequences for important social determinants of health including hours of work, gender equality and occupational health and safety.

There might be support for a stronger and more focused EU health policy. The 2019 institutional renewal – with new leaders in every top job, a new European Parliament without the grand coalition that had held since 1979 and a shift of focus away from austerity – offers a great deal of potential. Challenges such as populism, threats to the rule of law and popular dissatisfaction with many different issues all give leaders at the EU level opportunities to formulate more ambitious plans that can legitimate the EU by addressing major issues in popular and visible ways. Brexit, finally, will change the politics of the EU by removing one of its most consequential, and liberal, Member States.[3] There is scope to imagine something new and better in EU health policy: approaches that focus on health and well-being, on rule of law and protection of the vulnerable or on fulfilling the Pillar of Social Rights and SDGs are all possibilities. If the EU institutions were to declare that good health for all is a priority, this book has shown that it would be easy to both demonstrate EU success to date and identify powerful new policy options for the future. Likewise, a renewed commitment to well-being (Box 1.5) or to the European Pillar of Social Rights (section 3.5.3 and Box 3.5) could put the spotlight on existing EU achievements and potential policy options in health.

One way to emphasize the real and potential contribution of the EU to health is through the Sustainable Development Goals (Box 2.6). The European Union has a history of developing ambitious policy agendas as a way to give coherence and political force to its projects: the market integration of the Single Europe Act, the Lisbon Agenda, Europe 2020. The SDGs are somewhat different; they are goals agreed globally by the United Nations. While often associated with lower- and middle-income countries, they are also goals that no country has fully achieved, such as gender equality, good work and a sustainable environment,

---

3   Cylus J, Normand C, Figueras J, 2019. *Will population ageing spell the end of the welfare state? A review of evidence and policy options.* Copenhagen: WHO Regional Office for Europe, on behalf of the European Observatory on Health Systems and Policies; Greer SL, Laible J (eds.) (forthcoming). *The European Union After Brexit.* Manchester: Manchester University Press.

as well as good health and well-being. The EU's adoption of the SDGs (section 2.4), including as Semester goals, means that the fulfilment of the SDGs might be an opportunity to shape an agenda and narrative in which health becomes directly and indirectly a focus of EU policies. There is also abundant space for the EU to shape global health, including by replacing an increasingly withdrawn United States in many areas of standard-setting, reproductive health aid, and surveillance that are valuable.

The important thing to remember with all of these statements and agendas is that the EU, like any sophisticated political organization, can easily rebadge its existing and planned activity as part of a new agenda.[4] It is easy to be cynical, more so since anything as large and complex as the EU always has many agendas that might have little to do with one another – a frustration to any politician who seeks a coherent theme and agenda. The Juncker Commission sought to be "big on the big things and small on the small things", with health apparently a small thing. By the end of 2019 there was only one open legislative dossier in health and that was not moving quickly (HTA: section 4.6). Did that mean that EU policies affecting alcohol or food safety vanished? Of course not, and in fact DG SANTE continued to work on the many health issues discussed in chapter 3. Health lost strength as a constituency and a policy goal and its advocates in and outside the EU institutions have had to work to regain prominence over the last five years. Comparing the narrow mission letter sent to Commissioner Andriukaitis in 2014 (Appendix IV) to the activity discussed in this book shows the extent of their success. By the same token, though, declaring a new political priority that includes health will be an effective way to bring resources, energy and attention back.

6.3 Conclusion

The message of this book can ultimately be summarized in a few sentences. First, European Union health policy exists and affects both health and health systems. It is an awkward shape and has unusual features, procedures and priorities, but that is the case for most policy areas in any political system. This does not mean that there has ever been any pressure for a European health system, whether that is taken to mean financing of healthcare delivery, standard European entitlements or homogenization of the organizational features of healthcare systems. There is an almost complete absence of political or intellectual support for such an agenda.

Today, the EU is at something of a crossroads. It does much for health, in ways that stretch far beyond Article 168 and are not always regarded as health policy. It also misses many opportunities to improve health, whether through its weak

---

4   For example, European Commission (2019). *Reflection Paper towards a Sustainable Europe by 2030*. Brussels: European Commission.

system for regulating medical devices or through fiscal governance agendas that have been a threat to health budgets. There is public support for an EU that improves health, but little interest in EU healthcare services policy and resistance to some of the key EU regulatory policy tools for health. A decade of policy focused on exiting the financial crisis and promoting growth reshaped priorities and elaborated policy tools that can work across many fields. The legal space for EU action to improve health is enormous and by no means fully used, so much remains to be done.

6.4 Additional Reading

Anderson KM (2015). *Social Policy in the European Union*. Basingstoke: Palgrave Macmillan. A synthetic overview of social policy, including health, in the context of EU politics.

Greer SL, Kurzer P (eds.) (2013). *European Union Public Health Policies*. Abingdon: Routledge. Analyses of the politics of key EU public health policies, most of which have not changed much since 2013.

Hancher L, Sauter W (2012). *EU Competition and Internal Market Law in the Health Sector*. Oxford: Oxford University Press. A thorough legal treatment with a clear (pro-market) point of view, becoming dated.

Hervey TK, McHale J (2015). *European Union Health Law: Themes and Implications*. Cambridge: Cambridge University Press. The indispensable legal treatment of the topic, with strong policy and political understanding.

Hervey TK, Young CA, Bishop LE (eds.) (2017). *Research Handbook on EU Health Law and Policy*. Cheltenham: Edward Elgar Publishing. A collected volume with valuable and up-to-date analyses of important areas of law and policy.

Mossialos E et al. (eds.) (2010). *Health Governance in Europe*. Cambridge: Cambridge University Press. In large part dated, but in some areas the accounts remain the best syntheses available.

Appendices

I. Treaty articles relevant to health today in the Treaty on European Union

TITLE I

COMMON PROVISIONS

Article 2

The Union is founded on the values of respect for human dignity, freedom, democracy, equality, the rule of law and respect for human rights, including the rights of persons belonging to minorities. These values are common to the Member States in a society in which pluralism, non-discrimination, tolerance, justice, solidarity and equality between women and men prevail.

TITLE II

PROVISIONS ON DEMOCRATIC PRINCIPLES

Article 9

In all its activities, the Union shall observe the principle of the equality of its citizens, who shall receive equal attention from its institutions, bodies, offices and agencies. Every national of a Member State shall be a citizen of the Union. Citizenship of the Union shall be additional to and not replace national citizenship.

II. Selected articles relevant to health in the Treaty on the Functioning of the European Union (TFEU)

Source: Treaty on the Functioning of the European Union (Consolidated Version),[1] with reference to articles in the Treaty establishing the European Community (TEC) where relevant.

From   Part 1, Title 1, "Categories and Areas of Union Competence"

Article 4

1. The Union shall share competence with the Member States where the Treaties confer on it a competence which does not relate to the areas referred to in Articles 3 and 6.

2. Shared competence between the Union and the Member States applies in the following principal areas:

(a) internal market;

(b) social policy, for the aspects defined in this Treaty;

…

(k) common safety concerns in public health matters, for the aspects defined in this Treaty.

Article 6

The Union shall have competence to carry out actions to support, coordinate or supplement the actions of the Member States. The areas of such action shall, at European level, be:

(a) protection and improvement of human health; …

Article 9

In defining and implementing its policies and activities, the Union shall take into account requirements linked to the promotion of a high level of employment, the guarantee of adequate social protection, the fight against social exclusion, and a high level of education, training and protection of human health.

---

1   Council of the European Union (2012). Consolidated versions of the Treaty on European Union and the Treaty on the Functioning of the European Union. *Official Journal*, C 326:1–12.

From   Part Three, Title I, "The Internal Market"

Article 21 (ex Article 18 TEC)

1. Every citizen of the Union shall have the right to move and reside freely within the territory of the Member States, subject to the limitations and conditions laid down in the Treaties and by the measures adopted to give them effect.

2. If action by the Union should prove necessary to attain this objective and the Treaties have not provided the necessary powers, the European Parliament and the Council, acting in accordance with the ordinary legislative procedure, may adopt provisions with a view to facilitating the exercise of the rights referred to in paragraph 1.

3. For the same purposes as those referred to in paragraph 1 and if the Treaties have not provided the necessary powers, the Council, acting in accordance with a special legislative procedure, may adopt measures concerning social security or social protection. The Council shall act unanimously after consulting the European Parliament.

From   Part 3, Title II, "Free Movement of Goods"

Article 26 (ex Article 14 TEC)

1. The Union shall adopt measures with the aim of establishing or ensuring the functioning of the internal market, in accordance with the relevant provisions of the Treaties.

2. The internal market shall comprise an area without internal frontiers in which the free movement of goods, persons, services and capital is ensured in accordance with the provisions of the Treaties.

3. The Council, on a proposal from the Commission, shall determine the guidelines and conditions necessary to ensure balanced progress in all the sectors concerned.

Article 36 (ex Article 30 TEC)

The provisions of Articles 34 and 35 shall not preclude prohibitions or restrictions on imports, exports or goods in transit justified on grounds of public morality, public policy or public security; the protection of health and life of humans, animals or plants; the protection of national treasures possessing artistic, historic or archaeological value; or the protection of industrial and commercial property.

Such prohibitions or restrictions shall not, however, constitute a means of arbitrary discrimination or a disguised restriction on trade between Member States.

From   Part One: Principles – Title II: Provisions having general application

Article 15 (ex Article 255 TEC)

1. In order to promote good governance and ensure the participation of civil society, the Union institutions, bodies, offices and agencies shall conduct their work as openly as possible.

2. The European Parliament shall meet in public, as shall the Council when considering and voting on a draft legislative act.

3. Any citizen of the Union, and any natural or legal person residing or having its registered office in a Member State, shall have a right of access to documents of the Union institutions, bodies, offices and agencies, whatever their medium, subject to the principles and the conditions to be defined in accordance with this paragraph.

General principles and limits on grounds of public or private interest governing this right of access to documents shall be determined by the European Parliament and the Council, by means of regulations, acting in accordance with the ordinary legislative procedure.

Each institution, body, office or agency shall ensure that its proceedings are transparent and shall elaborate in its own Rules of Procedure specific provisions regarding access to its documents, in accordance with the regulations referred to in the second subparagraph.

The Court of Justice of the European Union, the European Central Bank and the European Investment Bank shall be subject to this paragraph only when exercising their administrative tasks.

The European Parliament and the Council shall ensure publication of the documents relating to the legislative procedures under the terms laid down by the regulations referred to in the second subparagraph.

Article 16 (ex Article 286 TEC)

1. Everyone has the right to the protection of personal data concerning them.

2. The European Parliament and the Council, acting in accordance with the ordinary legislative procedure, shall lay down the rules relating to the protection

of individuals with regard to the processing of personal data by Union institutions, bodies, offices and agencies, and by the Member States when carrying out activities which fall within the scope of Union law, and the rules relating to the free movement of such data. Compliance with these rules shall be subject to the control of independent authorities.

The rules adopted on the basis of this Article shall be without prejudice to the specific rules laid down in Article 39 of the Treaty on European Union.

From   Part 3, Title IV, "Free Movements of Persons, Services and Capital"

Article 48 (ex Article 42 TEC)

The European Parliament and the Council shall, acting in accordance with the ordinary legislative procedure, adopt such measures in the field of social security as are necessary to provide freedom of movement for workers; to this end, they shall make arrangements to secure for employed and self-employed migrant workers and their dependants:

(a) aggregation, for the purpose of acquiring and retaining the right to benefit and of calculating the amount of benefit, of all periods taken into account under the laws of the several countries;

(b) payment of benefits to persons resident in the territories of Member States.

Article 49 (ex Article 43 TEC)

Within the framework of the provisions set out below, restrictions on the freedom of establishment of nationals of a Member State in the territory of another Member State shall be prohibited. Such prohibition shall also apply to restrictions on the setting-up of agencies, branches or subsidiaries by nationals of any Member State established in the territory of another Member State.

Freedom of establishment shall include the right to take up and pursue activities as self-employed persons and to set up and manage undertakings, in particular companies or firms within the meaning of the second paragraph of Article 54, under the conditions laid down for its own nationals by the law of the country.

Article 50 (ex Article 44 TEC)

1. In order to attain freedom of establishment as regards a particular activity, the European Parliament and the Council, acting in accordance with the ordinary

legislative procedure and after consulting the Economic and Social Committee, shall act by means of directives.

2. The European Parliament, the Council and the Commission shall carry out the duties devolving upon them under the preceding provisions, in particular:

(a) by according, as a general rule, priority treatment to activities where freedom of establishment makes a particularly valuable contribution to the development of production and trade;

(b) by ensuring close cooperation between the competent authorities in the Member States in order to ascertain the particular situation within the Union of the various activities concerned;

(c) by abolishing those administrative procedures and practices, whether resulting from national legislation or from agreements previously concluded between Member States, the maintenance of which would form an obstacle to freedom of establishment;

(d) by ensuring that workers of one Member State employed in the territory of another Member State may remain in that territory for the purpose of taking up activities therein as self-employed persons, where they satisfy the conditions which they would be required to satisfy if they were entering that State at the time when they intended to take up such activities;

(e) by enabling a national of one Member State to acquire and use land and buildings situated in the territory of another Member State, in so far as this does not conflict with the principles laid down in Article 39(2);

(f) by effecting the progressive abolition of restrictions on freedom of establishment in every branch of activity under consideration, both as regards the conditions for setting up agencies, branches or subsidiaries in the territory of a Member State and as regards the subsidiaries in the territory of a Member State and as regards the conditions governing the entry of personnel belonging to the main establishment into managerial or supervisory posts in such agencies, branches or subsidiaries;

(g) by coordinating to the necessary extent the safeguards which, for the protection of the interests of members and others, are required by Member States of companies or firms within the meaning of the second paragraph of Article 54 with a view to making such safeguards equivalent throughout the Union;

(h) by satisfying themselves that the conditions of establishment are not distorted by aids granted by Member States.

Article 52 (ex Article 46 TEC)

1. The provisions of this Chapter and measures taken in pursuance thereof shall not prejudice the applicability of provisions laid down by law, regulation or administrative action providing for special treatment for foreign nationals on grounds of public policy, public security or public health.

2. The European Parliament and the Council shall, acting in accordance with the ordinary legislative procedure, issue directives for the coordination of the above mentioned provisions.

Article 56 (ex Article 49 TEC)

Within the framework of the provisions set out below, restrictions on freedom to provide services within the Union shall be prohibited in respect of nationals of Member States who are established in a Member State other than that of the person for whom the services are intended.

The European Parliament and the Council, acting in accordance with the ordinary legislative procedure, may extend the provisions of the Chapter to nationals of a third country who provide services and who are established within the Union.

Article 57 (ex Article 50 TEC)

Services shall be considered to be "services" within the meaning of the Treaties where they are normally provided for remuneration, in so far as they are not governed by the provisions relating to freedom of movement for goods, capital and persons.

"Services" shall in particular include:

(a) activities of an industrial character;

(b) activities of a commercial character;

(c) activities of craftsmen;

(d) activities of the professions.

Without prejudice to the provisions of the Chapter relating to the right of establishment, the person providing a service may, in order to do so, temporarily pursue his activity in the Member State where the service is provided, under the same conditions as are imposed by that State on its own nationals.

From   Title IV, Chapter 3, "Services"

Article 62 (ex Article 55 TEC)

The provisions of Articles 51 to 54 shall apply to the matters covered by this Chapter.

From   Part 3, Title VII, "Common Rules on Taxation, Competition and the Approximation of Laws"

Article 114 (ex Article 95 TEC)

1. Save where otherwise provided in the Treaties, the following provisions shall apply for the achievement of the objectives set out in Article 26. The European Parliament and the Council shall, acting in accordance with the ordinary legislative procedure and after consulting the Economic and Social Committee, adopt the measures for the approximation of the provisions laid down by law, regulation or administrative action in Member States which have as their object the establishment and functioning of the internal market.

. . .

3. The Commission, in its proposals envisaged in paragraph 1 concerning health, safety, environmental protection and consumer protection, will take as a base a high level of protection, taking account in particular of any new development based on scientific facts. Within their respective powers, the European Parliament and the Council will also seek to achieve this objective.

From Part 3, Title X, "Social Policy"

Article 151 (ex Article 136 TEC)

The Union and the Member States, having in mind fundamental social rights such as those set out in the European Social Charter signed at Turin on 18 October 1961 and in the 1989 Community Charter of the Fundamental Social Rights of Workers, shall have as their objectives the promotion of employment, improved living and working conditions, so as to make possible their harmonisation while the improvement is being maintained, proper social protection, dialogue between management and labour, the development of human resources with a view to lasting high employment and the combating of exclusion.

To this end the Union and the Member States shall implement measures which take account of the diverse forms of national practices, in particular in the field of contractual relations, and the need to maintain the competitiveness of the Union's economy.

They believe that such a development will ensue not only from the functioning of the internal market, which will favour the harmonisation of social systems, but also from the procedures provided for in the Treaties and from the approximation of provisions laid down by law, regulation or administrative action.

Article 153 (ex Article 137 TEC)

1. With a view to achieving the objectives of Article 151, the Union shall support and complement the activities of the Member States in the following fields:

(a) improvement in particular of the working environment to protect workers' health and safety;

(b) working conditions;

(c) social security and social protection of workers;

(d) protection of workers where their employment contract is terminated;

(e) the information and consultation of workers; EN C 83/114 Official Journal of the European Union, 30.3.2010

(f) representation and collective defence of the interests of workers and employers, including co-determination, subject to paragraph 5;

(g) conditions of employment for third-country nationals legally residing in Union territory;

(h) the integration of persons excluded from the labour market, without prejudice to Article 166;

(i) equality between men and women with regard to labour market opportunities and treatment at work;

(j) the combating of social exclusion;

(k) the modernisation of social protection systems without prejudice to point (c).

2. To this end, the European Parliament and the Council:

(a) may adopt measures designed to encourage cooperation between Member States through initiatives aimed at improving knowledge, developing exchanges of information and best practices, promoting innovative approaches and evaluating experiences, excluding any harmonisation of the laws and regulations of the Member States;

(b) may adopt, in the fields referred to in paragraph 1(a) to (i), by means of directives, minimum requirements for gradual implementation, having regard to the conditions and technical rules obtaining in each of the Member States. Such directives shall avoid imposing administrative, financial and legal constraints in a way which would hold back the creation and development of small and medium-sized undertakings.

The European Parliament and the Council shall act in accordance with the ordinary legislative procedure after consulting the Economic and Social Committee and the Committee of the Regions.

In the fields referred to in paragraph 1(c), (d), (f) and (g), the Council shall act unanimously, in accordance with a special legislative procedure, after consulting the European Parliament and the said Committees.

The Council, acting unanimously on a proposal from the Commission, after consulting the European Parliament, may decide to render the ordinary legislative procedure applicable to paragraph 1(d), (f) and (g).

3. A Member State may entrust management and labour, at their joint request, with the implementation of directives adopted pursuant to paragraph 2, or, where appropriate, with the implementation of a Council decision adopted in accordance with Article 155.

In this case, it shall ensure that, no later than the date on which a directive or a decision must be transposed or implemented, management and labour have introduced the necessary measures by agreement, the Member State concerned being required to take any necessary measure enabling it at any time to be in a position to guarantee the results imposed by that directive or that decision. EN 30.3.2010 Official Journal of the European Union C 83/115.

4. The provisions adopted pursuant to this Article:

- shall not affect the right of Member States to define the fundamental principles of their social security systems and must not significantly affect the financial equilibrium thereof,

- shall not prevent any Member State from maintaining or introducing more stringent protective measures compatible with the Treaties.

5. The provisions of this Article shall not apply to pay, the right of association, the right to strike or the right to impose lock-outs.

Article 156 (ex Article 140 TEC)

With a view to achieving the objectives of Article 151 and without prejudice to the other provisions of the Treaties, the Commission shall encourage cooperation between the Member States and facilitate the coordination of their action in all social policy fields under this Chapter, particularly in matters relating to:

- employment,

- labour law and working conditions,

- basic and advanced vocational training,

- social security,

- prevention of occupational accidents and diseases,

- occupational hygiene,

- the right of association and collective bargaining between employers and workers.

To this end, the Commission shall act in close contact with Member States by making studies, delivering opinions and arranging consultations both on problems arising at national level and on those of concern to international organisations, in particular initiatives aiming at the establishment of guidelines and indicators, the organisation of exchange of best practice, and the preparation of the necessary elements for periodic monitoring and evaluation. The European Parliament shall be kept fully informed.

Before delivering the opinions provided for in this Article, the Commission shall consult the Economic and Social Committee.

From   Title XIV, "Public Health"

Article 168 (ex Article 152 TEC)

1. A high level of human health protection shall be ensured in the definition and implementation of all Union policies and activities.

Union action, which shall complement national policies, shall be directed towards improving public health, preventing physical and mental illness and diseases, and obviating sources of danger to physical and mental health. Such action shall cover the fight against the major health scourges, by promoting research into their causes, their transmission and their prevention, as well as health information and education, and monitoring, early warning of and combating serious cross-border threats to health.

The Union shall complement the Member States' action in reducing drugs-related health damage, including information and prevention.

2. The Union shall encourage cooperation between the Member States in the areas referred to in this Article and, if necessary, lend support to their action. It shall in particular encourage cooperation between the Member States to improve the complementarity of their health services in cross-border areas.

Member States shall, in liaison with the Commission, coordinate among themselves their policies and programmes in the areas referred to in paragraph 1. The Commission may, in close contact with the Member States, take any useful initiative to promote such coordination, in particular initiatives aiming at the establishment of guidelines and indicators, the organisation of exchange of best practice, and the preparation of the necessary elements for periodic monitoring and evaluation. The European Parliament shall be kept fully informed.

3. The Union and the Member States shall foster cooperation with third countries and the competent international organisations in the sphere of public health.

4. By way of derogation from Article 2(5) and Article 6(a) and in accordance with Article 4(2)(k) the European Parliament and the Council, acting in accordance with the ordinary legislative procedure and after consulting the Economic and Social Committee and the Committee of the Regions, shall contribute to the achievement of the objectives referred to in this Article through adopting in order to meet common safety concerns:

(a) measures setting high standards of quality and safety of organs and substances of human origin, blood and blood derivatives; these measures shall not prevent any Member State from maintaining or introducing more stringent protective measures;

b) measures in the veterinary and phytosanitary fields which have as their direct objective the protection of public health;

(c) measures setting high standards of quality and safety for medicinal products and devices for medical use.

5. The European Parliament and the Council, acting in accordance with the ordinary legislative procedure and after consulting the Economic and Social Committee and the Committee of the Regions, may also adopt incentive measures designed to protect and improve human health and in particular to combat the major cross-border health scourges, measures concerning monitoring, early warning of and combating serious cross-border threats to health, and measures

which have as their direct objective the protection of public health regarding tobacco and the abuse of alcohol, excluding any harmonisation of the laws and regulations of the Member States.

6. The Council, on a proposal from the Commission, may also adopt recommendations for the purposes set out in this Article.

7. Union action shall respect the responsibilities of the Member States for the definition of their health policy and for the organisation and delivery of health services and medical care. The responsibilities of the Member States shall include the management of health services and medical care and the allocation of the resources assigned to them. The measures referred to in paragraph 4(a) shall not affect national provisions on the donation or medical use of organs and blood.

From Title XV, "Consumer Protection"

Article 169 (ex Article 153 TEC)

1. In order to promote the interests of consumers and to ensure a high level of consumer protection, the Union shall contribute to protecting the health, safety and economic interests of consumers, as well as to promoting their right to information, education and to organise themselves in order to safeguard their interests.

2. The Union shall contribute to the attainment of the objectives referred to in paragraph 1 through:

(a) measures adopted pursuant to Article 114 in the context of the completion of the internal market;

(b) measures which support, supplement and monitor the policy pursued by the Member States.

3. The European Parliament and the Council, acting in accordance with the ordinary legislative procedure and after consulting the Economic and Social Committee, shall adopt the measures referred to in paragraph 2(b).

4. Measures adopted pursuant to paragraph 3 shall not prevent any Member State from maintaining or introducing more stringent protective measures. Such measures must be compatible with the Treaties. The Commission shall be notified of them.

From Title XX, "Environment"

Article 191 (ex Article 174 TEC)

1. Union policy on the environment shall contribute to pursuit of the following objectives:

- preserving, protecting and improving the quality of the environment,

- protecting human health,

- prudent and rational utilisation of natural resources,

- promoting measures at international level to deal with regional or worldwide environmental problems, and in particular combating climate change.

2. Union policy on the environment shall aim at a high level of protection taking into account the diversity of situations in the various regions of the Union. It shall be based on the precautionary principle and on the principles that preventive action should be taken, that environmental damage should as a priority be rectified at source and that the polluter should pay.

In this context, harmonisation measures answering environmental protection requirements shall include, where appropriate, a safeguard clause allowing Member States to take provisional measures, for non-economic environmental reasons, subject to a procedure of inspection by the Union.

3. In preparing its policy on the environment, the Union shall take account of:

- available scientific and technical data,

- environmental conditions in the various regions of the Union,

- the potential benefits and costs of action or lack of action,

- the economic and social development of the Union as a whole and the balanced development of its regions.

4. Within their respective spheres of competence, the Union and the Member States shall cooperate with third countries and with the competent international organisations. The arrangements for Union cooperation may be the subject of agreements between the Union and the third parties concerned.

The previous subparagraph shall be without prejudice to Member States' competence to negotiate in international bodies and to conclude international agreements.

III. EU Charter of Fundamental Rights.
Article 35 – Health Care

Everyone has the right of access to preventive health care and the right to benefit from medical treatment under the conditions established by national laws and practices. A high level of human health protection shall be ensured in the definition and implementation of all Union policies and activities.

IV. Excerpt from Mission Letter from Commission President Jean-Claude Juncker to Vytenis P. Andriukaitis, 1 November 2014

You will be the Commissioner for Health and Food Safety. You will, in particular, contribute to projects steered and coordinated by the Vice-President for Jobs, Growth, Investment and Competitiveness As a rule, you will liaise closely with him also for other initiatives requiring a decision from the Commission.

The EU has a well-developed food safety policy with a rather complete and mature legal framework. Given that the Commission already exercises substantial responsibilities in these areas, the priority is to fulfil these tasks to the best effect. This is central to the interests of citizens, as well as to consumer 3 confidence in a sector of great economic importance for the EU. At this stage, the priority should be on modernising or simplifying the existing legislation, in line with our better regulation principles, and in close cooperation with the first Vice-President, in charge of Better Regulation, Interinstitutional Relations, the Rule of Law and the Charter of Fundamental Rights.

In the area of human health, the tasks given to the Commission under the Treaty are more limited. The specific exclusion of national health policy and of the management of health services illustrate the importance of respecting the rules on subsidiarity and proportionality. At the same time, the EU can clearly help Member States address the challenge of increased calls on health services and more complex technological choices at a time of intense pressure on public finances.

During our mandate, I would like you to focus on the following:

- Ensuring that the Commission is always ready to play its part in supporting the EU's capacity to deal with crisis situations in food safety or pandemics. • Working together with the Commissioner for Internal Market, Industry, Entrepreneurship and SMEs to jointly develop EU policies as regards medicines and pharmaceutical products while taking fully into account that medicines are not goods like any other.

- Within the first six months of the mandate, reviewing the existing decision-making process applied to genetically modified organisms (GMOs), in line with the Political Guidelines.

- Developing expertise on performance assessments of health systems, drawing lessons from recent experience, and from EU-funded research projects to build up country-specific and cross-country knowledge which can inform policies at national and European level. To the extent that it relates to the quality and productivity of the EU workforce, to the modernisation of social protection systems and to the quality and effectiveness of public expenditure, this expertise can also usefully inform the work of the European semester of economic policy coordination.

- Supporting the Commissioner for Humanitarian Aid and Crisis Management in his capacity as EU Ebola coordinator in his urgent work to further reinforce the EU Ebola response capacity.

V. Mission Letter to the Commissioner-designate for Health - Brussels, 10 September 2019

Ursula von der Leyen

President-elect of the European Commission

Mission letter

Brussels, 10 September 2019

Stella Kyriakides Commissioner-designate for Health

Dear Stella,

Earlier this year, the people of Europe made their voices heard in record numbers at the European elections. They presented us with a mission to be decisive and ambitious on the big issues of our time that are shaping the future of our society, economy and planet.

Changes in climate, digital technologies and geopolitics are already having a profound effect on the lives of Europeans. We are witnessing major shifts all the way from global power structures to local politics. While these transformations may be different in nature, we must show the same ambition and determination in our response. What we do now will determine what kind of world our children live in and will define Europe's place in the world.

Our job as the European Commission will be to lead, to grasp the opportunities and to tackle the challenges that these changes present, working hand in hand with people from across Europe and with the governments, parliaments and institutions that serve them.

This is the guiding principle behind my Political Guidelines for the next European Commission 2019-2024, which I presented to the European Parliament on 16 July 2019. I outlined six headline ambitions on which I want the European Commission's work to focus. These priorities are interlocking and are part of the same picture. In this spirit, I have put together a College in which we will all work, decide and deliver together.

An open and inclusive way of working

This approach reflects the open, inclusive and cooperative way of working that I will instil throughout the Commission, as well as in our relationships with others.

The College: One team

The European Commission functions on the **principle of collegiality**. This means we are one team: we all work together following a whole-of-government approach, we all have our say, we all decide collectively and we all take ownership of what is agreed.

To help us deliver on our ambitions and commitments, **I will empower eight Vice Presidents** to steer and coordinate thematic Commissioners' Groups on each of the Commission's priorities. They will be supported in this role by the Secretariat-General. All Commissioners will be in one or more Groups. The Commissioner for Budget and Administration will report directly to me.

Of the eight Vice-Presidents, the **three Executive Vice-Presidents** will have a dual function. As Vice-Presidents, they will lead a Commissioners' Group and be supported by the Secretariat-General. In addition, they will also manage a policy area and have a Directorate-General under their authority for this part of their job. One of the three Executives, First Vice-President Timmermans, will chair the College in my absence.

The High Representative/Vice-President will support me in coordinating the external dimension of all Commissioners' work. To ensure our external action becomes more strategic and coherent, it will be systematically discussed and decided on by the College. To support this, all services and Cabinets will prepare the external aspects of College meetings on a weekly basis, mirroring the process already in place for interinstitutional relations. This should also better align the internal and external aspects of our work. This will be a **'Geopolitical Commission'**.

I believe that we need to **speak and listen more to one another**, starting from within the Commission. College meetings will be places of open and honest discussion. As President I will set the agenda, but all College decisions will be taken collectively. In line with our commitment to fully digitalise the Commission and the need to use resources conscientiously, College meetings will be paperless and digital.

Each Commissioner will ensure the delivery of the **United Nations Sustainable Development Goals** within their policy area. The College as a whole will be responsible for the overall implementation of the Goals.

Interinstitutional relations and better policy making

Along with our close relations with the Council, I want to strengthen the Commission's **special partnership with the European Parliament**. This priority must cut through the work of each Member of the College, starting with myself.

I will expect you to ensure the European Parliament is regularly briefed, notably before major events and at key stages of international negotiations. In light of my support for a right of initiative for the Parliament, you should work closely with the relevant Committees, and be active and present during the preparation of resolutions requesting that the Commission legislate.

The more we build a consensus when designing policy, the quicker it can become law and make a difference to people's lives. This is why we need an **open and cooperative approach throughout the legislative process**, from policy design to final agreement. I will expect you to attend all political negotiations, known as trilogue meetings, with the other institutions.

We need to ensure that regulation is targeted, easy to comply with and does not add unnecessary regulatory burdens. The Commission must always have the leeway to act where needed. At the same time, we must send a clear signal to citizens that **our policies and proposals deliver and make life easier** for people and for businesses.

In this spirit, the Commission will develop a new instrument to deliver on a '**One In, One Out' principle**. Every legislative proposal creating new burdens should relieve people and businesses of an equivalent existing burden at EU level in the same policy area. We will also work with Member States to ensure that, when transposing EU legislation, they do not add unnecessary administrative burdens.

Proposals must be evidence based, widely consulted upon, subject to an impact assessment and reviewed by the independent Regulatory Scrutiny Board. You will ensure that they respect the principles of **proportionality and subsidiarity** and show the clear benefit of European action.

Given that any legislation is only as good as its implementation, I want you to **focus on the application and enforcement of EU law** within your field. You should provide support and continuous guidance to Member States on implementation, and be ready to take swift action if EU law is breached.

Bringing Europe closer to home

I want to **strengthen the links between people and the institutions that serve them**, to narrow the gap between expectation and reality and to communicate about what Europe is doing.

We must engage with all Europeans, not just those who live in the capitals or are knowledgeable about the European Union. I will expect you to **visit every Member State within the first half of our mandate** at the latest. You should meet regularly with national parliaments and take part in Citizens' Dialogues across our Union, notably as part of the Conference on the Future of Europe.

A stronger relationship with citizens starts with building trust and confidence. I will insist on the **highest levels of transparency and ethics** for the College as a whole. There can be no room for doubt about our behaviour or our integrity. The Code of Conduct for Commissioners sets out the standards and the rules to follow.

You will ensure budgetary spending represents value for taxpayers and follows the principles of sound financial management.

Making the most of our potential

The gender-balanced College I am presenting today makes good on my pledge to put together a Commission that is more representative and draws on all of our potential. This is a good start, but there is plenty more work to be done.

I expect you to **draw on all of Europe's talents** when it comes to setting up your own Cabinets. That means striking an appropriate balance in terms of gender, experience and geography.

The Commission should also lead by example when it comes to ensuring better representation and a diversity of voices in our public life. With this in mind, all public events organised by the Commission should aim to feature gender-balanced panels and a broad range of perspectives from across Europe.

Your mission

I would like to entrust you with the role of Commissioner for Health.

Europeans expect the peace of mind that comes with access to healthcare, safe food to eat and protection against epidemics and diseases. Europe has some of the world's highest standards on animal and plant health, as well as the most affordable, accessible and high-quality health systems to deliver on these expectations.

At the same time, we are becoming an older society and need more complex and expensive treatments. This brings into sharp focus the need to support the health sector and the professionals working within it, to invest in new technologies, to promote healthy lifestyles and to cooperate better within the EU.

Protecting and promoting public health

Your task over the next five years is to support Member States in constantly improving the quality and sustainability of their health systems. You should find ways to improve information, expertise and the exchange of best practices for the benefit of society as a whole.

- I want you to look at ways to help ensure Europe has the **supply of affordable medicines** to meet its needs. In doing so, you should support the European pharmaceutical industry to ensure that it remains an innovator and world leader.

- I want you to focus on the effective implementation of the new regulatory framework on **medical devices** to protect patients and ensure it addresses new and emerging challenges.

- We need to make the most of the potential of **e-health** to provide high-quality healthcare and reduce inequalities. I want you to work on the creation of a **European Health Data Space** to promote health-data exchange and support research on new preventive strategies, as well as on treatments, medicines, medical devices and outcomes. As part of this, you should ensure citizens have control over their own personal data.

- Many of today's epidemics are linked to the rise or return of highly infectious diseases. I want you to focus on the full implementation of the European One Health Action Plan against **Antimicrobial Resistance** and work with our international partners to advocate for a global agreement on the use of and access to antimicrobials.

- I want you to prioritise communication on **vaccination**, explaining the benefits and combating the myths, misconceptions and scepticism that surround the issue.

- I want you to put forward **Europe's Beating Cancer Plan** to support Member States to improve cancer prevention and care. This should propose actions to strengthen our approach at every key stage of the disease: prevention, diagnosis, treatment, life as a cancer survivor and palliative care. There should be a close link with the research mission on cancer in the future Horizon Europe programme.

Food safety and animal and plant health

Your work on food safety, animal welfare and plant health will play an important role in delivering on the European Green Deal.

- I want you to lead on a new **'Farm to Fork' strategy for sustainable food**. This will cover every step in the food chain from production to consumption, and feed into our circular economy objectives. It should combine regulation with communication and awareness campaigns and have full buy-in from local, regional and sectoral actors, as well as Member States and European institutions.

- As part of delivering on our **zero-pollution ambition** and 'Farm to Fork' strategy, I want you to work on protecting plant health, reducing dependency on **pesticides** and stimulating the take-up of low-risk and non-chemical alternatives. You should help protect citizens from exposure to **endocrine disruptors**.

- Part of your work will be to focus on **improving consumer information**, notably by looking at ways to address demands for more visible and complete information, especially on the health and sustainability of food products.

- **Animal health and welfare** is a moral, health and economic imperative. You will ensure Europe is equipped to prevent and fight against animal diseases that can be transmitted. You should also ensure the enforcement of animal welfare legislation, review our current strategy and promote European standards globally.

- I want you to focus on **the implementation and enforcement** of the extensive legislation in the areas of food safety and animal and plant health. Audits will be a crucial tool for this, notably to ensure that food imports meet our safety standards.

- You should work with the Member States to develop a **strategy with concrete measures against food fraud**, drawing on the work of the European Anti-Fraud Office in this area.

As a rule, you will work under the guidance of the Executive Vice-President for the European Green Deal on issues relating food safety, animal and plant health, and the Vice- President for Protecting our European Way of Life on public health matters. The Directorate-General for Health and Food Safety will support you in your work.

The way forward

The mission outlined above is not exhaustive or prescriptive. Other opportunities and challenges will no doubt appear over the course of the next five years. On all of these issues, I will ask you to work closely with me, and with other Members of the College.

Once there is more clarity, we should be ready to pave the way for an ambitious and strategic partnership with the United Kingdom.

I look forward to working closely together at what is an exciting and testing time for our Union. You can of course count on my full personal and political support ahead of your hearing at the European Parliament and throughout our mandate.

Yours sincerely,

Ursula von der Leyen
President-elect of the European Commission